IF IN DOUBT

An Anaesthetist's Story

Dr Keith Wilkinson

Published by New Generation Publishing in 2021

Copyright © Dr Keith Wilkinson 2021

First Edition

The author asserts the moral right under the Copyright, Designs and Patents Act 1988 to be identified as the author of this work.

All Rights reserved. No part of this publication may be reproduced, stored in a retrieval system or transmitted, in any form or by any means without the prior consent of the author, nor be otherwise circulated in any form of binding or cover other than that which it is published and without a similar condition being imposed on the subscquent purchaser.

ISBN
Paperback 978-1-80369-057-5
Ebook 978-1-8-369-065-0

www.newgeneration-publishing.com

New Generation Publishing

For our lovely grandchildren,
Zac, Marlie, Evie, Brooklyn, Kai, Rori and Rio.

Contents

FOREWORD 1
INTRODUCTION 3
CHAPTER 1: Crossroads 7
CHAPTER 2: Liverpool 18
CHAPTER 3: Fear 26
CHAPTER 4: Failure 35
CHAPTER 5: Finals 44
CHAPTER 6: Noble's 56
CHAPTER 7: Hurdles 75
CHAPTER 8: Newcastle 93
CHAPTER 9: Mistakes 112
CHAPTER 10: Clefts 127
CHAPTER 11: Hope 142
CHAPTER 12: Dilemmas 156
CHAPTER 13: Death 177
CHAPTER 14: Changes 194
ACKNOWLEDGEMENTS 212

FOREWORD

One of the many joys of a career in medicine is the friendships experienced on your professional journey. Unexpected friendships with people of all ages, and of many ethnicities, from around the world, whom one encounters by chance during years of hard toil. Some such friendships are long-lasting, working with the same colleagues for many years, but others are only transient and thus can be bittersweet. Hence it is always a delight to unexpectedly meet past colleagues again by chance, at professional meetings, or even on vacation. In such ways, my path has frequently crossed with Dr Wilkinson's over many years. Reminiscing is another aspect of a career in medicine that all of us enjoy when we suddenly meet a former colleague after a long time.

These pleasures especially apply to doctors who have trained with you. To see them mature and go on to contribute, in many different ways, to the broad spectrum of medicine, be it clinically, educationally, academically or in hospital administration, is enormously satisfying. Every medical school, and every professor, is proud of their successful protégés, in whatever walk of life they have become established.

Dr Keith Wilkinson is one such protégé. From the beginning of his career in anaesthesia in Liverpool, it was clear that this trainee was an honourable and hard-working man of sharp intellect, with no delusions of grandeur. Many of us in the Liverpool School of Anaesthesia would have liked Keith to work with us at consultant level and urged him to do so. But he had emotional ties both to the North East of England and to the Isle of Man, that he describes in this book. We were sorry when he left us but are proud of

If In Doubt

the contribution he went on to make at consultant level in the Isle of Man for exactly thirty years. We also recognise fully the international charitable work he has carried out using his anaesthetic expertise in the most extreme of circumstances. All of this demanding work has covered a wide spectrum of clinical specialities, but Dr Wilkinson had been well trained for it as this book exemplifies. Health care in the United Kingdom would be even safer if all clinicians practised to the same high standards of anaesthesia as Dr Wilkinson.

As I read this book, I was surprised to recognise many of the same emotions Dr Wilkinson describes as I have experienced along my clinical journey. I too longed to be a doctor from an early age, had a strong and supportive family, and was always returning to the intensive care unit to find out how my patients were progressing. Dr Wilkinson is at all times honest about the challenges he has faced throughout his career and is, in true British fashion, often self-denigrating. But his story is well worth reading by all those considering a career in medicine, and especially one in anaesthesia. I am certain all his hospital colleagues in the Isle of Man will be interested to read this book, too – do they remember any of the clinical scenarios? – as will many of his non-medical friends on the island.

Dr Wilkinson and I have both been fortunate that we have retained sufficient good health to fulfil our dreams. I wish him well in his retirement and trust he will continue to write such monographs for which he is now becoming well-recognised. He is an absolute credit to the medical profession, and especially to the speciality of anaesthesia. I thank him for all the work he has done for humanity.

Jennifer M Hunter MBE
University of Liverpool, England

INTRODUCTION

Have you ever thought how astonishing it is that you can remain safe, pain free and most of all, *alive,* even during the deadliest of medical procedures? Have you ever wondered exactly what it takes to make sure you're properly anaesthetised? Or feared what might go wrong?

Whether you're a curious lay person considering a career in medicine, or even thinking of training in anaesthesia, I wrote this book for you.

If In Doubt draws on stories taken from the sharp end of what has always been, to me, the most fascinating of all the medical specialties. Anaesthesia didn't just change modern surgical approaches, it *created* them, allowing surgical intervention to go where it could never go before. Yet it is also a speciality steeped in mystery; few people ever learn what really goes on behind the scenes when they're lying unconscious on the operating table.

I wrote If In Doubt to show you. In it I intersperse real-life medical triumphs and tragedies, taken from a career in anaesthetics that spanned thirty-seven years, with easy-to-digest medical explanations. Exactly thirty of these years were spent as a consultant in a small island hospital where I was in the unique position of having to know every area of anaesthetics and every ward. From the operating theatre to palliative care at the hospice. From the challenges of ICU and life-threatening major trauma, to the orthopaedic, gynaecology, paediatric and general surgery wards, I worked everywhere. I could be preparing patients to be air-lifted to Liverpool one moment then administering epidurals for caesarean sections in the obstetric unit the next. I never missed a day off work sick and every day was different. I loved each one.

I hope you enjoy this book. Many of the opinions I offer throughout these pages are my own. Other medical professionals might disagree. That is medicine. It is a profession that is constantly evolving with ongoing research and new developments in treatment. When several doctors are involved in a patient's care, opinions can vary widely on treatment options. What is vital though, is that more than anything, each doctor wants what is best for the patient. I know I did, and I hope If In Doubt gives the reader an entertaining and informative insight into anaesthetics, the best career I could have ever chosen.

All author proceeds from the sale of this book will be donated to the NSPCC.

If In Doubt

My Mam was dead. I was convinced of it. At three and a half this was to become my earliest memory, the tears I cried for her as vivid now as they were sixty-one years ago. She'd gone into hospital for the birth of my brother, and it would be four long weeks before I'd see her again. When she did finally come home, bringing my new brother with her, I'd hidden, weeping, behind the settee, refusing to come out. I remember Mam had been too weak to climb the stairs, so Dad had set up a bed for her in the sitting room. It was like this that I'd slept safely tucked beside her for the next few weeks, happy once more.

Years later I'd found out how close she'd come to death and learnt how she'd only been saved by an emergency hysterectomy following her caesarean section. Doctors had saved my mam. That was it. I wanted to be one.

If In Doubt

CHAPTER 1

Crossroads

Dumble. Surely it had to be one of the best surnames ever. He was my technical drawing and woodwork teacher at Chester-le-Street, near Durham. The bookcase he'd helped me make during my first year at the school in 1968 had been on my bedroom wall ever since, holding my treasured collection of true crime and bird books. He was also the school's careers teacher and I needed to talk to him now.

I was about to embark on my second term in sixth form, and, as 'Bart', my form tutor and Head of PE, Mr Hunter, had pointed out just a few weeks earlier, my future at the school was looking bleak.

It had been a cruel summation. Handing out our school reports, he'd told a few of us that we had effectively wasted our time for the previous four months, as well as that of our teachers.

To say we had learned nothing, however, was unfair and not entirely correct. Perhaps I had learnt little, if anything, of maths, chemistry and physics, my three A-levels. It was also true I had scored only 27 % in my end of term physics exam. This had resulted in me being kicked out of that subject and, instead, I was due to start A-level art after Christmas.

On the other hand, through many hours spent in the library, diligently, quietly – hidden from prying eyes, behind a bookcase, my friends and I had been learning skills of a different kind. Cards.

At the end of that first term, the four of us who played regularly considered ourselves budding gamblers. One or two had even wondered whether we might make a living from blackjack or three-card brag.

Then, payback time arrived. Mr Hunter had looked at me, shook his head and said,

'Do you actually understand the work?' I stared back and said nothing. The silence that followed had seemed to last forever, until, under the gaze of my classmates, my teacher had turned away, his lack of confidence in me still evident in his shaking head.

Later, on the way home, I had read his comments about my abysmal performance during that term.

'...but with his present attitude towards work his standard of attainment is so poor that he has now reached a crossroads.'

It was harsh, but deep down I knew it was fair. Something had to change. Now Christmas break was over, and I'd been thinking about nothing else. It was time to speak to Mr Dumble.

For as long as I could remember, I'd wanted to be a doctor. Being the sixties, without the access to the information we have now, my direct experience of the profession was limited. I'd spent three nights in hospital after an ENT procedure when I was seven and was familiar with fictional characters such as Dr Kildare, who seemed to have an impressive impact on my mother and sister. My only experience beyond that, but one that left a lasting impression, was when my mother almost died.

It was only many years later when it dawned on me that the doctors had saved her life, and now, here I was, my own long-held dream of one day becoming one myself rapidly fading.

Mr Dumble's solution to the problem was simply to 'lower my sights.' It was the first time in my life I had ever heard that expression, as we sat together alone in the technical drawing classroom. He asked if I had considered an alternative career as a medical lab technician, pointing out that with nine O-levels, I wouldn't need A-levels for this type of job. It was an interesting proposition. My dad had been in the Royal Navy during the Second World War and now and then I had considered following in his footsteps. I wondered if a position as a medical lab technician in the Navy might be the answer.

A few days later therefore saw me at the Royal Navy careers office in Newcastle, taking tests in general knowledge, maths and English, which I passed with ease. Then it was off on the long journey to the Royal Hospital Haslar in Gosport, near Portsmouth, for an interview which took place in one of the hospital labs with a middle-aged man in a white coat. I was clearly qualified and was offered the job immediately, but then he looked up, leant forward, and suddenly said,

'What do you really want to do?'

I told him what I really wanted was to be a doctor but didn't feel I was clever enough to achieve the grades. In any case, I'd failed miserably in physics and an art A-level certainly wasn't going to impress any medical school. His response took me by surprise – that perhaps I should think about knuckling down at school and give being a doctor my best shot.

On my way home, a brief detour in London, my first time in the capital, gave me time to think. With my interest in true crime, I naturally headed via the underground to Madame Tussauds to see the Chamber of Horrors and its waxwork figures of notorious killers. I then spent the entire four-hour journey home thinking about what we'd discussed at my interview. By the time I'd reached Durham, I'd formulated a plan, and the following morning I went straight from school assembly to find my form tutor.

Mr Hunter's name was a perfect fit, and I felt apprehensive as he strode towards me, a panther approaching its victim. He was a keen sportsman, and there was no doubting this as he stood facing me in his usual fern-green tracksuit and white trainers, complete with obligatory white stripes.

I looked at him, took a deep breath, then announced I wanted to make a serious attempt at getting grades good enough to get into medical school. It was a big move. I would need to stay on at school an extra year, and it would also be necessary to make some changes to my subjects.

Mr Hunter looked sceptical about this, but he wished me luck, saying,

'You need to prove to yourself and to me how committed you are to seeing this through.'

It was a start, now I just had to convince everybody else.

Luck was on my side. Next up was the biology teacher, who agreed I could start A-level biology with the class below me when their course started after the summer break. He also said I could join in my own year's course whenever I was able to. In addition, he wanted me to take the O-level in that subject at the same time, reckoning I could pass that in a further six months or so.

Last on my list of teachers was Mr Poulter, my maths teacher and Deputy Head. I asked him if, as well as carrying on with maths, I could also take further maths. I honestly didn't think I'd ever pass and in this I was right, but I wanted to do it in order to help my ordinary maths A-level. Having essentially done no schoolwork at all for the previous six months, I was now about to start studying A-levels in maths, further maths, biology, chemistry and art, as well as O-level biology.

My friends could hardly believe what they were witnessing. We'd often meet up for a few drinks in the pub at night, even though we were underage. All that stopped. My mother managed to get an old table for my bedroom to use as a desk and over the next few days, I got into a rhythm that went something like this:

After getting in from school I'd have a meal then lie down for a short sleep, maybe an hour or so. Around seven o'clock I'd go up to my room and start studying, mainly maths, as that was my weakest subject. Around midnight, my mother would bring me up a cup of hot chocolate and ask if I'd be going to bed soon. I always said 'yes,' but never did. It would often be around two o'clock when I'd fall asleep. At half past eight, I'd be off to catch the bus to school and my day's ritual would start all over again.

I was studying like my life depended on it. On top of my general homework, I'd asked Mr Poulter to lend me books. From these I'd pick random questions on calculus, differentiation and integration and put them in for marking too. One day he was handing out the homework in class. When he came to me, he said it was disappointing to see some of my classmates hadn't submitted any answers, particularly when I'd done about three times more work than I'd been asked to do. I got some stick later for being a 'swot,' but they all knew why I was doing it. It was the only way I had a chance of getting top grades.

I was so ambitious to succeed that my determination occasionally overshadowed my responsibilities. In October my sister got married, and I was their best man. By then, my studying was ingrained. After she'd set off for her honeymoon with my new brother-in-law, everyone else came back to our house. Unthinkingly, I automatically went up to my room to study. My dad had to come to remind me that my relatives were there and wanted to see me. I remember feeling ashamed of my ignorance and selfishness.

Around this time, my mother also started a part-time job as a cleaner in a hospital, St Margaret's in Durham. It was only years later I realised she'd only done this so my parents would have a little extra money to help me through my five years of medical school. Everyone was taking my goal seriously.

A few months later, I said goodbye to my classmates after their A-levels, then, after the summer break, I was back in the class below my own for my final year, ready to begin the long-awaited process of preparing for medical school.

As well as intense study, part of this preparation was to be the application procedure for medical school. This, in itself, was a straightforward process, and not unlike applying for any university course – pick five and place them in order of preference. Teachers then gave predicted grades, which helped the universities decide who to offer places to. Unfortunately, this meant I had a problem. It came in the form of my chemistry teacher, Mr Williams, or 'Splutterguts' as he was affectionately known – due to an unfortunate habit of sometimes spitting when he spoke. I knew he would have predicted something like a grade D. If this really was the case, I was doomed. No medical school would give a provisional offer with that sort of prediction.

Splutterguts was a tricky character in general. A few years earlier, I'd been on the receiving end of a beating from him for talking during a lesson. Without warning, he'd lost control, dragged me out to the front of the class by my hair, and punched me several times in the head with his fist, the first joint of his middle finger sticking out slightly so it would hurt that little bit more. I had felt I was seeing stars like a cartoon character as I was dragged by the collar of my blazer and pushed hard out of the classroom.

Later, I'd proudly let my classmates feel the three or four bumps. Later I witnessed others receive the same, or even worse treatment. Now I had to get him to believe in me. In spite of everything I still had a lot of respect for him as a teacher; maybe I'd deserved my punishment a few years earlier. I realised I needed his help and that was all that mattered now. There were very few interviews for medical school in those days. Being head boy or girl, or captain of a school team might have helped sway the balance in a student's favour. Mainly though, it was academic ability that won the day and my chemistry teacher had hinted on a few occasions that medical school was, he felt, 'a bit out of my reach.'

Then something interesting occurred. One morning, in the library, I picked up the Oxford University prospectus and saw that Oxford required application to a specific college. In the small print I read that if a candidate listed Christ Church first on their UCCA application form, they were automatically guaranteed an interview. It was perfect.

If In Doubt

I knew full well I'd never get in but decided I'd try anyway – just so I could see Mr Williams' reaction when I told him I'd been offered an interview not just at any medical school, but Oxford itself. He couldn't possibly have known that I'd get an interview just for putting Christ Church as my first choice, and so, though I had no real wish to go to Oxford, I applied. It would be an experience and I'd get to have a look around Oxford for a few days, all paid for too.

Splutterguts tried hard but failed to hide his surprise when I told him my good news and mumbled some vague words of congratulations. I mumbled some words of my own, one beginning with 'F' as I walked away, smiling.

In early December 1975, I went by train to Oxford. As it was Christmas and most students had left for the break, I was given a student's flat for the two nights. After putting on my suit, I headed for a sherry, wine and cheese reception. There were boys from the Westminster Public School in London wearing long jackets and funny ties, showing us around and serving drinks. As far as I could see, they were just there to show off, bragging about what they were up to, who they knew and what their dads did and earned, amongst other things. I had no interest in what they were saying and decided there and then I wouldn't go to Oxford even if I was offered a place.

After a few minutes, I slipped away and changed back into my jeans and new black leather bomber jacket, an early Christmas present from my mother. I then headed for the nearest bar, The Bear, where I stayed for the next five hours or so. The following morning, my sore head and I were rudely awakened to the sound of someone moving around in the living room. When I opened the bedroom door, I was surprised to see a man in a suit, looking under the settee.

'I'm looking for your shoes,' he said. 'You are supposed to leave them outside your door at night so I can polish them.' I told him not to worry and they were fine as they were.

This world of shoe-polishing butlers and magnificent Tudor halls of long tables, stained glass windows, and oak-panelled walls hung with portraits, was a different world to the one I knew.

Over the course of the next few days, there were to be several interviews. Finally, in one, I was asked what sort of books I liked to read. I'm not sure what they hoped my answer might be, perhaps Dickens, Orwell or Hemingway, but I am fairly certain they could never have predicted my answer:

'I only read about true crime, true murder,' I said. My interviewer looked taken aback, replying,

'That's a funny thing to be reading!'

'I don't agree,' I'd answered. 'There's nothing funny about murder, to me it's fascinating,' This had been my parting shot. If I hadn't already done myself out of a place at Oxford, I think I'd done it now.

Back home, a few days later, I received the letter I knew was coming. I'd failed to gain a place there. Sod them, I thought, I wouldn't have gone anyway. I hoped that Mr Williams had been sweating over the last few weeks, worrying in case I had been successful. I never told him I wasn't.

One by one over the next few weeks, I was turned down by the other four universities on my list. I now knew that unless I could get into a university after the A-level results came out in August, I would be going nowhere that year. The clearing system, which allowed for those without a conditional offer to secure that of another who hadn't made the grades, was now my only hope. First, of course, I had to get good enough grades myself – and only As or Bs would do for a place at medical school.

The exams came and went, and I felt confident I'd done enough. Now came the waiting game.

In the meantime, my sister had managed to get me a job as a nursing auxiliary at a mental health facility, Earls House Hospital, near Durham where she worked as a medical secretary. I soon settled into the job, helping to look after around thirty residents in roughly twelve family units, or 'villas,' for patients aged between five and seventy.

Some housed only children, one elderly men and another elderly women, and so on. At first, I dreaded certain parts of the job, especially taking them to the toilet and bathing some of them, but within a few days I had adjusted and was enjoying the work.

At the end of July 1976, in the middle of the hottest summer on record, I had a fortnight's holiday with the rest of my family and my aunt and uncle, and cousin and her boyfriend, in a cottage in Lochcarron on the west coast of Scotland, near Skye, before returning to my job. When the results came through, I was absolutely delighted to have been awarded an A in chemistry, A in biology, B in maths and a fail, as expected, in further maths. I was enjoying the nursing job so much by now, however, that I'd secretly already made up my mind – university could wait for another year.

My mother had different ideas, of course, as mothers often do. Reluctantly, I therefore rang one or two universities only to find they were full. Then, one afternoon, I tried Liverpool. It was a pivotal moment, and one I will never forget.

The secretary there told me that with my grades, if I'd called a few hours earlier, I'd have got their last place, and that if I applied again, and put Liverpool first on my UCCA form, it was almost guaranteed I'd get in. That was it, I didn't need to try anywhere else, there would be no medical school for me that year, and in December of the same year, 1976, I finally received what I'd worked so hard to achieve – a firm offer from Liverpool University. I'd done it. I was in.

For the rest of the academic year, I therefore relaxed and enjoyed every minute of my job at Earls House Hospital. It was rewarding and humbling, and I met and worked with some lovely people, both residents and nursing staff. I also felt confident that this year was giving me a head start for medical school.

I'd been presented with a three-pound book voucher for my A-level results. With the knowledge that our first anatomy dissection in Liverpool would be on the arm, I'd used it to purchase a book on the subject, diligently working my way through the intricacies of the muscles, nerves and bones in preparation. My work at the villas had also given me a good grounding in antipsychotics and antidepressants, as many residents were on these medications. I would read about these drugs, or ask the nurses and psychiatrists to explain them to me, learning about their mechanism of action and side effects.

Some of the residents with severe learning difficulties had extremely rare syndromes such as Tuberous sclerosis and Cornelia de Lange syndrome. Tuberous sclerosis is a genetic condition where non-malignant tumours develop throughout the body in the brain, skin, heart and kidneys and is associated with severe learning disabilities. Cornelia de Lange syndrome is a developmental condition resulting in dwarfism, severe learning difficulties and often severe bony abnormalities of limbs, hands and fingers.

Four years later, during my twelve-week paediatric attachment at Alder Hey Hospital in my third year of medical school training, my consultant paediatrician tutors would be amazed when I told them I knew all about these conditions. Many of the patients were also epileptic. I must have seen at least fifty seizures during my year there, so I'd learnt the side effects of the anti-epileptic drugs.

On Monday October 3rd 1977, I was finally due to start as a medical student. I could hardly wait. There was just one last thing I needed to do.

After the summer break, in early September, I returned to my old school to thank my headmaster Mr Driscoll, and his deputy Mr Poulter. The latter I especially wanted to thank for his encouragement and help in getting my B grade in maths. After they had both wished me well, I headed off towards the chemistry lab. This was the moment I'd been looking forward to more than anything. I was going to let Splutterguts know I was going to medical school, and it was no thanks to him. I wanted to see his reaction.

Sadly, I was in for a disappointment. When I arrived there, the classroom was empty. I was puzzled, and went to the next classroom in the science block to ask where Mr Williams might be.

'He's retired,' I was told.

I never saw him again.

CHAPTER 2

Liverpool

I can still remember when I first heard them on Radio Luxembourg in 1963, *From me to you*, The Beatles' first number one hit. Although I was only six, it had an impact on me I've never forgotten. In my opinion, it was the best music out there, and fifty-seven years later, I still consider it to be some of the greatest music ever produced.

Throughout my life, Paul McCartney and John Lennon have been my favourite musicians. *Penny Lane*, *Strawberry Fields*, the list goes on, and every time I hear them it takes me back to my childhood: Durham Swimming Club, endless sunny days in the garden, looking for birds' nests, and playing football in the schoolyard with a pair of rolled up gloves (footballs were banned due to an unfortunate incident with the headmaster's window). The Beatles' music was my childhood in song. It therefore seemed fitting that I was about to train to be a doctor in Liverpool.

Thursday 29th September 1977 was my twenty-first birthday, and in four days' time I would start my medical studies. With a September birthday, and having dropped back a year in sixth form before working for a year, I was three years older than many of my soon-to-be fellow medical students. I travelled by train on the Saturday and settled into my room in Dale Hall on the Carnatic Site near Aigburth, about three miles from the centre.

That first morning, Monday October 3rd, was spent getting a feel for the university. I did what all students do – filled out forms, joined the Students' Union. I also checked out the campus and the bookshop, Parry Books. At lunchtime I had a few beers with the friends I'd met in the halls of residence on my first night in the students' bar, The Augustus John, or 'The AJ' as it was known.

If In Doubt

Then the big moment finally arrived. It was a tradition that all new medical students were welcomed by the Professor of Anatomy, Professor Harris, in the ancient oak-panelled lecture theatre at 2pm on their first day. The steeply rising rows of wooden benches were packed with eager students and I instinctively walked up to the back row. As this was already full, I took a seat in the next row down. I knew no one, but little groups were talking excitedly and the noise from the multiple combined conversations in the small theatre was deafening. There was a sense of anticipation and an eagerness to get started with our training, anything to make us doctors that little bit sooner.

When Professor Harris walked onto the stage, white-coated and white-haired, tall and erect, a respectful silence descended on the lecture theatre. He started by reminding us how fortunate we were to be there. For each one of us, there were ten disappointed young men and women who would have given anything to swap places. Their futures were uncertain, but ours, if we worked hard, were guaranteed to be the best futures anyone could wish for – rewarding and interesting. We had a responsibility, he continued, to live up to the opportunity we'd been given and we needed to think now and then of the sacrifices our parents had made to give us that chance of a fulfilling career as a doctor. We were lucky, and we should always remember that.

For a few brief moments, I was enthralled by the message he was trying to convey, feeling honoured and proud to be there. That special moment, however, was about to be ruined.

At first, I wasn't sure if I was hearing things. Giggling, whispering, more sniggering.

'Shut up, for fuck's sake!' I recognised the accents as Scouse; they sounded just like the Beatles. 'Honest to God,' they continued. 'If he doesn't fucking shut up…' More tittering.

Irritated, I cautiously turned around to identify the source. Two faces stared blankly back at me, silent now. Their shabby appearance only served to heighten my irritation on what was, in my eyes, an important day. Despite their momentary silence, they seemed to question 'What's your problem?' Keen to avoid a confrontation, I therefore focused my attention back on the Professor, determined to bask in the significance of our achievement. The disapproving comments recommenced almost instantly and I was outraged.

What were they thinking? Did they have no respect? Did they not understand that this was a special day for me, and the other one hundred and forty-odd students in the lecture theatre, a day we'd never forget? It took only a few seconds more for the truth to hit me. In the build up to our big day, I'd almost forgotten one simple fact. This was Liverpool.

Looking back, it was the perfect start to my career as a doctor. They were Scousers. No respect for authority, cynical, suspicious, with an instinctive refusal to accept being told what to do – unless there was very good reason to do it; an ingrained inability to tolerate any form of perceived 'showing off' or pomposity. In a way, it was easy for me to accept this attitude because Geordies were the same. Lovely and honest, caring people, like the Liverpudlians, but also not used to being told what to do. Any self-respecting Scouser or Geordie would have behaved the same – medical student, docker. It didn't matter what their vocation, they were Scousers and proud. Of course, at the time, after only two days in the city, I didn't yet realise this. Now, after having lived there for nine years during medical school then during my anaesthetic training, I look back and smile, because I know it was a great introduction to Liverpool life. I was going to fit right in.

After the Professor's talk we had another medical school tradition to face, the dissection room. On that first afternoon, we crammed the stairs from the lecture theatre and the hall outside, anxiously waiting to see how we would react to the forty cadavers awaiting our amateurish attempts to learn about the structure of their bodies through careful dissection.

The corpses had once been human beings who had requested their bodies be donated to 'medical science.' As we entered the room, there was a musty scent in the air, reminding me of an unclean changing room at a swimming pool. It was the odour of formalin and decay.

The bodies, covered in white sheets, brought with them a new wave of silence, as all one hundred and fifty students shuffled into the room. Most couldn't resist the temptation, lifting the crisp sheet just enough to peek at the body nearest to where they stood.

Jostling for space around the metal tables on which the corpses lay, Professor Harris appeared once again at the front. He reminded us of the need to always remember that these corpses had been fathers or mothers, brothers or sisters and grandparents. At all times we were to treat their bodies with respect.

Through careful dissection, we were to learn the points of insertion and origin of muscles onto the bones, the course of the nerves supplying those muscles, the arteries and veins, internal organs, heart and lungs and most difficult to learn of all, the brain. He explained that there would be four students to each body, in one or two cases three. We'd be instructed at the start of each session what to look for during dissection by demonstrators. These were qualified doctors, usually Senior House Officers (SHOs), who were training to be surgeons or Accident and Emergency doctors. Some had taken six months out of their clinical work to do this. They were paid a similar wage to the one they'd have received for working in their own specialties.

Once we got started, the demonstrators would wander between the tables, stopping here and there to discuss what we were doing and see if we had any queries. There were usually three or four demonstrators for each session. There were two of these, lasting about three hours on a Monday and Thursday afternoons, although we were allowed to go in and out if we needed to do a little extra dissection as long as we got permission from the demonstrator.

Professor Harris himself would be in and out and we noticed he often gravitated towards tables where pretty girls were working. He hardly ever bothered us, which suited us just fine. He was tall and slim with a rigid military posture – his white coat invariably buttoned up to the top as if to limit any unwanted lapses from his acquired textbook authoritative stance. Wearing a red and white spotted bow tie, he habitually approached each group with his hands clasped behind his back, peering over the top of wire-rimmed half-spectacles as if carrying out his own meticulous dissection of the student doctors who stood before him.

The first part of the body we looked at was the arm, then the leg, head and neck, chest and finally the abdomen and pelvis. Each part took around ten weeks to dissect and study, and at the end of each there would be an oral exam, or 'viva.' We had to arrange with a demonstrator a suitable time and place to do this – it could be in a quiet part of the dissection room, or even just at the table itself. Our group opted for the pub, the Prince of Wales. Here, we'd meet at lunchtimes, paying, as was tradition, for the demonstrator's drinks, whilst they'd ask each of us questions. It lasted for around an hour, but inevitably, after the viva was over and the demonstrator had left, we'd stay in the pub for a few hours. Our success would be marked in the viva in a book kept in the dissection room. If anyone failed, they had to repeat the task until they passed, before being allowed to move on to the next part of the body.

Within a few weeks, naturally, little cliques developed – groups of students who would have coffee together in the student union cafe, drink together in the bar, or sit close to each other in the lecture theatres.

For the first five terms, around twenty months, we studied three subjects: anatomy, physiology and biochemistry. It was all lectures, small tutorial groups, lab work and dissection. My little group consisted of around eight core members and four or five hangers-on, who would come and go.

In some gangs in the US there are initiation ceremonies, and any would-be gangster has to prove he is worthy, perhaps by taking on other gang members. The rules differ for different gangs, but some would say if he could give a good account of himself in a fist fight against three gang members for thirty seconds and still be standing, or had at least landed some good punches, he was in.

Our rules didn't involve any violence, of course, and were never made explicitly clear to the members. The first rule none of us could influence anyway, and this was that your surname had to fall at the end of the alphabet. Russell, Saunders, Shearer, Walker, Weighill, Wells, Whiteside, Wilkinson. Most of the initial bonding took place as we huddled around the cadavers during dissection and the tables were allocated in alphabetical order, as was the physiology and biochemistry lab seating.

The second, and maybe the most important rule, was that you had to enjoy drinking pints, and lots of them. This included drinking during most lunchtime breaks in the nearby Stag's Head, the Old Fort, The William or the Students' Union bar.

Another one involved the use of a briefcase. Anyone seen carrying one of these pretentious items was considered a snob. To be 'one of us,' it was customary to transport all books and other necessary (though limited) possessions, in a carrier bag, preferably a plain white one. Finally, any student who either sat at the front of the lecture theatres on a regular basis, or, even worse, routinely put up their hand, would also be shunned for being an intolerable show-off. These were unwritten rules. No one wrote them because they didn't exist, but that didn't matter. To us, or certainly to me, they were a part of our identity and no exceptions were allowed.

Once in the gang it was clear to each of us that we had to continue in the same vein. Buying a briefcase further into our course would be met with scorn. For me, this has carried on throughout my life as demonstrated by the following anecdote, which happened ten years later.

On December 1st 1987, a Monday, I started my first day in Newcastle as a Senior Registrar. At the time we were staying with my parents whilst our new house purchase was going through. The previous Saturday, my mother and my wife had been shopping in Durham. When they came back, they gave me a present for starting the new job – an Antler briefcase. It had cost one hundred and fifty pounds. I pretended I liked it and glanced at my dad, my hero, a little embarrassed. I'd also followed more unwritten rules unknowingly set by him, copying his likes and dislikes. Never wear a hat, no matter what the weather. Never wear a raincoat or an overcoat. Never wear gloves, no matter how cold it might be. Don't even think about carrying an umbrella.

On my first morning, I'd set off early on the drive to the General Hospital in Newcastle. I got out of the car, took hold of the briefcase, locked the car door, and walked about ten yards before stopping. A vision of my dad, disapprovingly shaking his head at the sight of me carrying such a symbol of snobbery, had stopped me in my tracks. What was I thinking? Without hesitation, I headed back to the car, placed the briefcase on the back seat, took out its sole contents, my ham sandwich, and left it there never to be used by me again. It just didn't feel right.

I hid this briefcase in the boot of my car for a long time, then in the back of a wardrobe. Years later, however, it eventually found a use. I gave it to my youngest daughter when she was about eight, and she'd proudly carry her sheet music in it to her singing and piano lessons.

As with my A-level studies, even though I was making the most of the student lifestyle, I had quickly established a strict routine of studying each night before joining my friends later in one of the nearby pubs, the Rose and Crown in Mossley Hill, or the Aigburth Arms. Friday night was different. It was my night off from everything; I'd go out on my own but would usually end up joining a group of Scousers, invariably ending the evening in a night club until the early hours.

After a few months some of the other students would join me on my Friday night adventures. The time for poring over anatomy books, lab experiments, dissecting the entire body, learning by heart hundreds of chemical reactions and enzyme chains, drinking and ensuring we all stuck to our gang rules, was coming to an end.

After the first year in Dale Hall, I'd taken the decision to live on my own in a bedsit in Oxton, Birkenhead, in order to guarantee the peace and quiet I needed to study. I'd often not bother travelling in for lectures, instead studying on my own in the bedsit. The groundwork was done, and I passed my anatomy, physiology and biochemistry exams which signalled the end of the preclinical part of the course. The rest of the five years of my training were to consist of much anticipated clinical work – which would test our potential as real doctors, facing real live patients, who, unlike the cadavers, might notice our inexperience.

CHAPTER 3

Fear

It was May 1979. The first day of the clinical part of our five-year degree course had arrived, and everyone was apprehensive.

We all wanted to be doctors, even those habitual hand-raisers who seemed only to want to prove they knew the theory. None of us wanted to be biochemists or clinical physiologists, or even medical lab technicians. Nowadays, with modern medical student education, clinical work and patient contact starts immediately. For us, only after a year and a half into medical school, it was time to face real patients for the first time, no-nonsense Scousers too, who by then we all knew wouldn't take kindly to any bullshitting or showing off. It was terrifying.

Being frightened wasn't helpful, and meant we were probably in no position to be honest. There would be the scorn and stern words from our doctor tutors to worry about if we weren't up to scratch, also the potential for ridicule from the ward nurses, especially the ward sisters, and fear of embarrassing ourselves in front of our fellow students. It would be even worse if they were in our own little gang. We'd never hear the end of it. It was a minefield. Any shame and we'd have to live with it for the rest of our training, maybe even the rest of our lives, but there was no alternative. We were going to have to do our best and hopefully not upset too many doctors, nurses, or patients along the way.

Ward 8X and 8Y in the Royal Liverpool Hospital, 8am on a Monday morning. We had been allocated to our firms, groups of usually eight to twelve students that would rotate around the various medical specialities for the next three years.

If In Doubt

I was in a group with nine others, and our first attachment was medicine, a massive speciality within a vast range of specialities, including everything from general practice to genito-urinary medicine, pathology, psychiatry – the list goes on. Undergraduate students received a basic grounding in each area, then branched out only after graduation. It was a sobering thought. One day we would all have to decide where our future lay, then work out how to achieve it. There would be many sacrifices, on-calls, studying for exams, stress. It was going to be difficult from now on, whichever way we looked at it.

As we gathered, a game of spot the student doctor would have been easy. There we stood in our freshly ironed white coats with neatly pressed shirts and ties. Our stethoscopes were folded and safely hooked over the top of the pocket, a little status symbol that could be just about seen by patients and nurses. We'd been told we needed to get one from a shop close to the Royal and it was a big moment for me when I bought mine. Some of us also had a medical book in the opposite pocket. Later I was amused to discover that some of my student colleagues only ironed the front of the collar and about six inches of the top-front of their shirts, either side of the buttons – the only part visible when they wore a white coat.

Either way, we were suitably equipped, and ready for whatever we had to face, or so we thought. Our first job was to be briefed in the tutorial room by a Senior House Officer (SHO) in Medicine. He explained the protocol we should follow when we saw our first patients. Be smart, courteous and introduce ourselves; let the patient know we were students but explain we were under the strict supervision of doctors, so they had no reason to worry. Be polite, and at the same time try to appear confident and remember that however fearful we might be, the patient was more even so.

He then ran though the age-old technique for talking to patients: history, examination and order investigations.

Based on these we were to try to come up with a diagnosis, or at least a provisional diagnosis, then start treatment.

Next, each of us were allocated four patients and told we had the rest of the morning to talk to them and obtain an understanding of their symptoms and a full medical history. We were then to use our stethoscopes to examine their hearts and chests, check their blood pressure, examine the abdomen, and anything else that was necessary. After this, we were expected to formulate a tentative diagnosis. Later, our tutor would take the whole group back on the ward. The student who had seen the patient was to present the history, examination and provisional diagnosis to the group for discussion.

Our tutor left us, saying he'd be back after lunch so we could have time to complete a ward round, and that we'd meet back up to discuss the patients we'd seen. After he went, we sat in silence. This was it, the moment we'd waited for, but we were riddled with nerves. Feigning confidence, I got up and wandered casually onto the ward before casually wandering back out again without speaking to anyone and went back to the tutorial room. Biding my time, I had a coffee and admitted to myself I was delaying the inevitable. If I wanted to be a doctor, then eventually, at some point during the rest of my career, which might last forty years, I was going to have to speak to a patient. It was time to grow a pair. But this new-found backbone quickly crumbled as I dismissed the thought and sat back down, just as someone asked,

'How many patients have you seen?' It was a girl who wasn't in our little clique. I looked at her with a nervous smile.

'None,' I replied. 'How many have you seen?'

'Same as you,' she said. 'None. To be honest, I'm having second thoughts about this whole thing.' She seemed on the verge of tears.

'Tell you what,' I said. 'We're both in the same boat and we're all nervous. Let's just go for it and meet back here in an hour, what do you think? We can have a coffee and tell each other how it went?'

'Okay,' she said, her voice a little shaky. 'But if it doesn't work out, I think I'm getting out of all of this. Maybe I'm just not cut out for it.'

I went first. A young girl, about twenty years old, lay in bed with abdominal pain. She looked as if there was little wrong with her. Asking whether she'd had diarrhoea, whether she might be pregnant, and about her periods, was difficult. With each question I was terrified I might overstep the mark. I had visions of being grilled by a General Medical Council (GMC) disciplinary panel as to why I felt it necessary to ask a twenty-year-old virgin such pointless questions. Was I going to be the youngest ever doctor to be struck off the medical register?

Of course, I needn't have worried. She understood I was a student and that this was a big part in our preparation to ensure we had the experience and the confidence to communicate with any patient. Without that, I would be unable to give my patients my best care. It was a valuable lesson for the rest of my career.

As our confidence grew, everything became more enjoyable. One day our SHO tutor said he had organised a special ward teaching session. He had four patients for us, each of whom knew they would die in the next few weeks.

We went to the bedside of each of the four and it was explained that we were students but might learn something from each of their stories. Throughout the rest of my career, I have never come across the courage and honesty I witnessed that day. They were so matter of fact and brave about their imminent deaths. Some even cracked a few jokes. One said everything had happened so quickly he couldn't believe the situation he had found himself in, but at least he'd had the time to organise his affairs.

None of them appeared upset or cried. They would have been asked in advance if they minded talking to us, so would have had a little time to prepare. Even so, it still struck me that they had all accepted the inevitable, and though one or two were afraid of dying alone or in pain, their main concern was that they die as peacefully as possible.

It was a humbling experience. Throughout my career, the thing I have feared more than anything is dying while suffering from unrelieved dyspnoea. Dyspnoea is the medical term for the sensation of struggling to breathe and asthmatics know it well. The heavy smoker with severe COPD (chronic obstructive pulmonary disease) also lives with it on a daily basis, with intermittent exacerbations when they develop a chest infection. During these periods they may be prescribed antibiotics or a temporary increase in the dose of their regular steroid tablets to tide them over.

Dying patients sometimes develop sudden heart failure, often because of myocardial infarction: a heart attack. They can present with acute pulmonary congestion. This is when the left side of the heart can't pump out the blood arriving from the right side, having first passed through the lungs. This creates a build-up of pressure in the capillaries in the lungs, resulting in fluid from the blood leaking into the tissues around the microscopic air sacs, or the alveoli. The result of this is that the lungs become stiff and heavy, like a pair of sponges dipped in water, and it is accompanied by the need to gasp for breath.

In severe cases, frank pulmonary oedema occurs, when fluid fills the alveoli and enters the smaller of the larger airways and pours out the mouth in a pink froth. There are few more satisfying medical emergencies to treat in medicine than this condition. Sitting the patient upright, giving oxygen, intravenous diamorphine (heroin) and an intravenous diuretic to increase fluid lost from the body via the kidneys, combined with other drugs to reduce the pressure in the lung capillaries, often results in a fast and dramatic improvement. Diamorphine is the perfect drug in this setting, relieving the dyspnoea, having a euphoric and sedative effect, relieving the pain from the aching breathing muscles, and helping to reduce the pressure.

Talking to patients about their fears surrounding imminent death was a learning experience, and one I have never forgotten over a forty-year period. It also taught me the importance of speaking to dying patients with honesty and integrity. Like many doctors of my age now, I have seen hundreds of dying or dead patients, and spoken to their relatives. In giving the worst news they could ever hear I've never said, 'He passed away' or 'I'm sorry, she didn't make it.' They died. I have never seen any point in avoiding that word during discussions with patients or their loved ones. Using a different phrase won't make things sound less tragic.

I feel there needs to be a more honest approach towards some patients who are at high risk of imminent death. DNARs (Do Not Attempt Resuscitation orders), are now a common part of the management of all patients in hospital, not only medical patients. Through these, a discussion with the patient can reveal their own wishes as to whether they would like to be resuscitated in the event of their heart stopping. To me, this has been one of the major improvements in the care of some patients during my career. It avoids futile and very traumatic attempts to restart the heart when it is inappropriate. It also takes away the need for the often difficult decision to start resuscitation when someone collapses suddenly, as this decision will already have been made.

The rest of our medical attachment was spent seeing and presenting numerous patients on the wards, attending clinics and ward rounds, tutorials and lectures. It was an eye opener. Many medical conditions like diabetes, chronic lung disease, rheumatoid arthritis and ischaemic heart disease are incurable. All the physician and the GP can do is optimise treatment to control the patient's illness and try to limit the progress of the disease so they can enjoy as good a quality of life as possible for as long as possible. With drug treatment there is often a fine balance between relieving symptoms and slowing down the progression of the disease and avoiding unpleasant side effects. A physician and a GP might also see the same patient on a regular basis throughout their entire career, possibly even thirty-five or forty years. What if I didn't like them, or they didn't like me?

In the last week of the attachment, we went out with the two consultants who had been teaching us for the traditional firm dinner, a custom repeated several times during the remainder of the course. By then I had decided. Medicine wasn't black and white, but a million shades of grey. I preferred black and white so that was it, medicine wasn't for me.

We were now two years down with three to go, and after the summer break we were straight into our new attachment, three months of surgery. The training was similar. We learnt how to take a good history, assisted in theatre, and sat in clinics watching the consultant interact with patients. We also had small tutorial groups and the usual nine o'clock lecture in the Duncan Building adjoining the Royal. These could be on medicine or surgery, but I rarely attended as I found it more productive to glance at notes taken by a friend and read up about the subject later in my bedsit. After the lectures, students would head off to their respective hospitals in Liverpool.

With surgery, we started to be on call at night, shadowing the house officer, a doctor in his first year after qualification. This is known as a doctor's pre-registration year, when his or her name goes to the GMC to be placed on a provisional register. Only after six months of medicine and six of surgery, and if it was deemed by your consultants that you had done a reasonable job, did you go onto the full register. Then it was time for the big decision – whether to enter GP training, the most common choice, or whether to begin the journey up the ladder, with the hope of eventually obtaining a consultant post in hospital. Ranking grades went as follows:

If In Doubt

SHO for one or two years, registrar for three or four years, senior registrar for three years, then finally, consultant. The best jobs for registrars and senior registrars (SRs) were rotational posts, where the whole three years were mapped out for the doctor, with either three, or six-month blocks in different hospitals. During the registrar job there was the hurdle of the postgraduate exam. This had to be passed before a senior registrar job became a possibility. For the medics this was the MRCP (Member of the Royal College of Physicians). In surgery, the equivalent was FRCS (Fellow of the Royal College of Surgeons).

Anaesthesia at that time had as their qualification FFARCS (Fellowship of the Faculty of Anaesthetists in the Royal College of Surgeons). Years later the anaesthetists managed to obtain their own college in London and the qualification today is FRCA (Fellow of the Royal College of Anaesthetists). But for me, all of this was a long way off.

During the surgical attachment we learnt how to suture wounds in theatre and the A&E department. We gained experience in taking blood and inserting intravenous cannulas. We'd see all the emergency patients with the house officer, slowly learning how to elicit a patient's history so we could follow the trail of clues to achieve a provisional diagnosis. We were detectives in white coats. If a patient's complaint was abdominal pain, we needed to know as much as possible. As an example of how thorough we had to be, here is a list of the types of questions we were expected to ask.

Where was the pain? In a specific spot, or generalised? Could the patient point to it? How and when did it come on, suddenly or gradually, and could they describe the pain? Did it ache or burn? Was it sharp, gripey, colicky, or constant? Was it improving or worsening, and did they feel ill? What made it worse – coughing or straining? Had there been any change in bowel habit, diarrhoea or constipation or any bleeding from the anus or blood mixed in with the stool? Had there been a sensation of having to open the bowels only to produce small amounts of faeces or a sudden onset of having to open the bowels, tenesmus? Had there been any weight loss, nausea or vomiting?

The sequence went like this: history, examination, investigations such as blood tests, X-rays then finally a provisional diagnosis or diagnoses. The most common of these for acute abdominal complaints were appendicitis, bowel obstruction, pancreatitis, peritonitis, often caused by a perforated ulcer in the stomach or the first part of the small bowel, the duodenum. Bleeding from the stomach or oesophagus often leads to the vomiting of blood, or haematemesis.

The most difficult part of our detective work, however, was deciding if and when an operation would be required. It was a huge responsibility. If things went smoothly and the patient made a good recovery, all would be well. When post-surgery complications developed, usually through no fault of the surgeon, it might be a different story. A complaint from the patient or their relatives might then follow, bringing with it associated worry and stress for the surgeon. To me it seemed a bit of a thankless task. At the end of the attachment, I'd therefore made another decision. I ticked it off the list. As with medicine, surgery wasn't for me.

CHAPTER 4

Failure

I'd always wanted to go to New York. There was something about the skyscrapers, the Statue of Liberty and the mix of cultures in Manhattan. I'd read travel brochures and books about it when I was at school and never missed an episode of *Kojak*, the fictional detective who worked the streets of the Big Apple in the mid-70s.

In March 1980, at the start of the Easter break, I decided to go and flew with Freddie Laker's Skytrain on a Jumbo Jet from Gatwick – my first time on a plane. I spent the entire journey standing at a bar at the rear of the cabin talking to a middle-aged man who was going there on business, and a very pretty girl, Sophie, who was on her way home to Harlem. I drank so much that when I went through Immigration at JFK airport, the officer couldn't read my writing. I had to sit in a room with ten or so others until I was able to write legibly. Some of these appeared very dodgy to me and they probably thought I looked the same.

'You're all set,' the Immigration Officer eventually said, smiling slightly as they stamped my passport after my second attempt at writing. I then left the airport and checked into a cheap hotel near Washington Square Park and, during the next few days, walked everywhere around Manhattan. Over the Brooklyn Bridge, to Central Park, the Empire State Building and the World Trade Centre.

I went on a boat trip around Manhattan that passed close to Liberty Island, and wandered through Chinatown and Little Italy. The sheer size of the buildings had a weird effect on me, and I lost any real sense of distance. I'd start to walk thinking the building I was headed to didn't seem that far away. After half an hour or so I'd still not be anywhere near it. When I looked at a scale map, I realised I was walking twelve to fifteen miles a day, maybe more. Apart from an educational cruise to Iceland and Norway when I was thirteen, I'd never been abroad.

A few weeks later I was back in Liverpool and things were getting serious. The medical degree consisted of two main parts. The Final MB, Part 1, was taken at the end of the third year. For us, this meant June, just a couple of months away. Leading up to these exams, which were in pharmacology, pathology and microbiology, I therefore decided to stay with my brother, Kevin, who was a chef in a hotel in Kendal, the Woolpack. I took my books with me. I reasoned I'd be away from my friends and be less tempted to go out at night rather than study. Spending almost three weeks there, I'd study all day in his room while he was working. As I travelled back to Liverpool on the train, I felt I'd done enough. I was wrong.

I failed pathology and only just passed the other two subjects. This was the first exam I'd failed. I'd passed the First MB – anatomy, biochemistry and physiology at the end of the preclinical part of the course. It came as a shock to fail such an important one now, three years into my five-year course. The pressure was on. I'd have to re-sit and pass the exam at the beginning of September, the start of my fourth year. If I failed again, it could mean the end of medical school for me. One of our group, my friend Chas, failed all three exams so he was in a far more serious position.

I thought back to my Royal Navy interview and how that had made me realise the only way I was going to get anywhere was through hard work. This was another wake-up call, and though I'd been looking forward to a nice summer break, I knew now that I would need to study instead. I had no other option. Next time, I had to pass. As I also needed to earn some money, I'd arranged to do some work as a lab technician in Durham during my six-week summer break. By an amazing coincidence, there was a pathologist working close by and she helped me with my studies.

I'd spend my coffee and lunch breaks talking to her and would ask her to question me to find weak areas I needed to read up on. She'd put interesting histology slides in her microscope for me to view and she'd test me, to see if I could identify them. This would be part of my exam. Normal tissues like stomach, pancreas, tongue and rare malignant tumours such as gliomas, found in the brain and melanoma, in skin. At night I'd go for a few pints but always had a book with me. I knew my mam was very worried and I was determined I couldn't let her or myself down again.

By this point I'd realised I'd totally underestimated the amount of studying I needed to do. I thought by missing out on lectures I could easily do the work from books, but I'd been wrong. I'd been lucky not to fail all three like Chas. When the end of the summer finally came, I had to go back to Liverpool a week early with the others who had failed exams as the re-sits took place before the rest of the students returned and year four started.

I managed to get a room in the doctors' residence next to the Royal and had a week to prepare. Chas was also staying there. We decided we had to do everything we could to ensure we passed. If we failed again, we could be out and neither of us really knew what else we would do if that happened. We therefore studied all day and relaxed in the evenings, and when the exams came I felt confident I'd done enough preparation. I had. I passed. So did Chas, in all three exams. We were back in business.

After this there followed three months of homelessness. That period was to be our paediatric attachment and I'd managed to get a room at Alder Hey for the entire time. I therefore decided to save on rent and left my bedsit in Birkenhead at the start of the summer. I stayed in a room in the hospital, with four of the twelve weeks spent living in accommodation at Leighton Hospital, Crewe, Whiston, and the Countess of Chester Hospital.

During this time, we were shown how to examine babies and older children, and learnt about illnesses in children of all ages on ward rounds and in clinics. Once a week I'd attend a clinic in Myrtle Street in the town centre where children with congenital heart disease were seen and operated on. Today much of the work of a cardiologist involves using an ultrasound probe to visualise the heart and its valves. At that time, though, the stethoscope carried far more importance than it does now.

We became skilled at diagnosing abnormalities through hours spent listening to heart murmurs caused by the blood swirling through the narrowed or leaking valves. We also went into the operating theatre at Myrtle Street where we watched heart operations. It was incredible to see the surgeon carrying out a life-saving operation on a baby's heart the size of a strawberry.

It was towards the end of this placement, at eight o'clock in the morning on December 8th 1980, that my friend and fellow trainee, Neil Russell, knocked on the door of my room at Alder Hey. He had some bad news. One of our musical heroes, John Lennon, was dead at forty, murdered in New York City.

Neil was a Beatles fan too, and ever since I was about six the Beatles had been my favourite musicians. My dad had been humming *From me to you* as he cooked breakfast or made a cup of tea for seventeen years, since its release. Being a student then in Liverpool and going past Penny Lane, Strawberry Fields, and the site of the Cavern Club, all made my student years even more enjoyable. I was where they had been, walking the same streets and drinking in the same pubs. I couldn't possibly be studying medicine in a better place.

The night he died the two of us went to the site of the Cavern Club where it had all started. There were messages and flowers there, the whole city was in mourning. From there we made our way to a restaurant for the traditional firm dinner with the consultant who had been responsible

If In Doubt

for our placement over the last twelve weeks at Alder Hey. The meal was a celebration of our latest placement, but it was a sad night for both of us, and for millions of others around the world.

A few weeks later, after the Christmas break, it was back to work and time for a few weeks in A&E at Walton Hospital. This was followed by a very important part of our course, twelve weeks in obstetrics and gynaecology, six weeks in each specialty. Four of us each had a room for the duration of the obstetric part of the course in Oxford Street Maternity Hospital in Liverpool. Coincidentally, John Lennon had been born there, and four years later our first daughter, Emma, would be born there too. For this part of the course, we had to help the midwives look after women in labour. Each of us had to be there for ten deliveries. These had to be verified by the midwives.

To me, childbirth was the most horrific thing I'd ever seen in my life. Screaming women, blood everywhere. Some babies were born after long and difficult labours and needed resuscitation to get them breathing. If a baby's head became stuck during labour, metal forceps would be used and it appeared to us the head might actually come off. The baby might be decapitated. We hardly dared look in case that happened, though of course it never did.

The hard-as-nails midwives didn't seem to be like other nurses we'd seen in other hospitals. Those nurses seemed to be nice, caring and sympathetic and wanted to do everything they could to help their patients. It appeared there was no time for any of that here. We realised it was probably an illusion, but to us they didn't seem to care about the pain, or anything else for that matter. There was no question that they were in charge of the patient's care and what they said went. They worked in a very busy and extremely stressful environment and simply couldn't allow themselves to deviate from a well-trodden path that led to the safe delivery of a healthy baby. A mistake or wrong decision could mean a dead or brain-damaged baby. Or a dead mother. We treated them with respect and they were always kind to us and taught us a lot.

As part of our studies, we had to write up six case histories of interesting patients we'd seen in clinics and during ward rounds. These would be marked and contribute to our final score in the final exams for this subject. Any of these cases could be discussed in our viva assessment at the end of the course.

Much of our teaching during this time took place during ward rounds with the consultants and the senior registrars. Professor Beasley was one of our tutors. We learnt how to examine a pregnant lady's abdomen and how to assess the size, gestational age in weeks, and the position of the fetus.

Knowing the position of the baby, the fetus, becomes important as the end of pregnancy approaches. The head usually becomes 'engaged' in the pelvis and starts to descend leading up to the start of labour. We learned how to examine the lower part of the abdomen and determine how much of the head was engaged. This was described as if the head was divided into fifths. If most of the head could be felt in the lower abdomen the head would be approximately one-fifth engaged. If only a small part could be felt it might be four-fifths engaged. The usual position is head-down, so this is the part that will be born first. The widest part of the head is about three-fifths so if it is three-fifths engaged no serious problems would be expected for the birth.

With a breech position the baby lies so that the head is high in the uterus and the baby's bottom will be born first. This increases the risk of complications during delivery. At that time many women with a breech presentation went through normal labour but a large study suggested a caesarean section is safer for the baby. Today, almost all of these patients have a caesarean section. As part of our training, we would also scrub up and assist during caesarean sections.

If In Doubt

During our earlier surgery attachments and in A&E we'd learnt to infiltrate local anaesthetic into wounds and suture them. Now we gained more experience in suturing episiotomies. An episiotomy is a cut made through the perineum and posterior wall of the vagina to enlarge the opening for the baby to be delivered through. In some patients a tear of the perineum, the muscular area between the vagina and anus, might occur so the cut is made to prevent this and allow a more controlled delivery.

Each night we'd take turns holding the bleep so we could be contacted if there were any imminent deliveries. One night I was in the Cambridge pub a few yards from the hospital, still in my white coat and enjoying a soft drink while the others were having a few beers, when my turn finally came. It was March 1981, and *That's Entertainment* by the Jam was blasting out the jukebox, a big hit at the time. After my bleep went off I rang the hospital on the payphone in the bar, and was told they were looking for me for a delivery.

I felt slightly guilty walking in and taking over from the trainee midwife to deliver the baby within fifteen minutes of arriving, all under the supervision of the midwives. The trainee midwife had been involved in the labour all day and needed to get in her own set number of deliveries. I'd walked in at the last minute to claim it for myself. There never seemed to be any hard feelings though, and I think the trainee midwives knew we felt bad. The fact was we had to demonstrate we had been involved in ten deliveries. That was one down, only nine to go.

One night while we were in the middle of the attachment the four of us went to a nightclub, The Razzamataz, 'The Raz' as it was better known. There I noticed a couple of lads glancing over. They seemed to be talking about us and none of us had seen them before. We left the club about one o'clock to walk back to the hospital, about half a mile away.

What happened next was so fast we had no time to react. Neil and Paul were walking in front, Euan and I behind, when the two lads we'd seen in the club ran past. They turned in front of Neil and Paul, punched them in the face once then ran off. My two friends both fell to the ground but were fully conscious and not badly hurt.

Instinctively, I took off after them and was gaining on them when after half a mile or so a police car pulled up alongside me. I explained what had happened and they told me to get in and radioed to other cars and the two were soon caught. We went back to where it had happened. The other three got into the car and we headed to the police station so we could give statements.

Suddenly, I felt sick and one of the policemen told me if I was I'd have to clean it up myself. To me it seemed they were blaming us for what had happened, and when we arrived at the station I got into an argument with the officer over his attitude. I was immediately arrested and taken to the Main Bridewell just off Dale Street, now the Caro Hotel. The first policeman went in but the other stayed outside for a few seconds and challenged me to a fight. Although I'd had a few drinks I knew now I needed to stay calm and not move, or I'd be in even serious trouble. I said nothing.

Once inside, I was told to empty my pockets then put in a large cell. It was about two thirty in the morning by now, and there were about eight men in there. I sat down on a wooden bench. After a few minutes one of them wandered over and sat next to me. He was huge, wearing jeans and a blood-stained white t-shirt. His head was shaved, and tattoos covered his muscular arms. He asked what I was in for and I told him. Then he asked what I did for a living. When I told him, the reaction was not what I had been expecting.

'Fucking hell!' he said. 'You're going to be a doctor?'

I nodded.

This was followed by silence as he looked me up and down then turned to the others.

'This lad's a fucking doctor! He shouldn't be in with the likes of us. If any of you bastards go near him I'll fucking kill you! The fucking police. Bastards. Cunts, the lot of them!' There was silence again.

I had to smile, even though the realisation of what was happening was dawning on me. If the Dean of the medical school found out I'd be in serious trouble. My new bodyguard told me to plead not guilty, which I did at about ten o'clock in the magistrate's court later that morning. I was released at lunchtime and the other three were waiting for me outside. Paul had a black eye. I later changed my plea to guilty of being drunk and disorderly, and several months later I went to the same magistrates' court in Dale Street. Luckily for me no one in authority at the university had heard about the case, but I was about to get a nasty surprise.

I was led into the dock and looked across to the three magistrates. The middle one was a consultant physician from the Royal and I'd spent twelve weeks on his firm two years earlier. He'd recently retired. He'd even given me a letter explaining how pleased he was with my work and wished me well for the future. I'd taken it home to show my mam and she'd kept it and proudly showed it to her friends and my aunties.

In the end I was fined eighteen pounds and he asked how I intended to pay. I had the money in my pocket so I paid there and then. When I told the others that night they thought it was hilarious. A few weeks later back home for Christmas, in a pub one night with my dad and his mates, they couldn't stop laughing. I was lucky I heard no more about it as I was fairly sure he must have recognised me. If he did he could have potentially ended my career by informing the Dean and it was good of him to keep our little secret.

CHAPTER 5

Finals

After the sometimes exciting and interesting obstetrics came six weeks of gynaecology. None of us had the faintest interest in this part of the course but it was important in terms of the final exams. There would be written papers, a viva exam and the dreaded vaginal examination with a speculum. Part of our course involved us attending clinics at Fazakerley Hospital, now Aintree. During one of these Paul, Neil and myself were there. Mr Benson, the consultant, was due to retire soon and we followed him in and out of various rooms as he saw and examined patients.

He explained to one patient, a young lady who was about thirty, that we were students and that she needed a vaginal examination and one of us was about to do this under his supervision. She was complaining of pain during intercourse and heavy blood loss during menstruation.

We'd been shown how to do this on our first day of the attachment and it was something all medical students dreaded. Stories circulated about students failing finals because they hurt the patient during a speculum examination. We were never sure if they were true but they terrified us. It certainly worried me.

A speculum is a metal instrument used to carry out the procedure and there were two types, Cusco's and Sims. For the actual exam itself we could choose whichever one we preferred. I always chose the Sims as to me it was much easier to insert and, more importantly, there was less risk of causing pain – and potentially failing the final exam in obstetrics and gynaecology.

I was amazed when Neil bravely stepped forward to volunteer and sat on a stool in front of the patient's exposed perineum. Paul and I stood idly behind him, pretending to be taking a keen interest and listened as the consultant explained to the patient that Neil would need to insert a speculum into her vagina so he could inspect her cervix.

So far so good. I felt quite proud in a way that Neil had saved us from this awkward task and thought that the least we could do to repay him was to watch and learn. I'd buy him a pint later as a thank you. She was quite relaxed and Neil proceeded in his task, talking to us and the consultant as he did so.

'The perineum appears healthy, vaginal mucosa is normal and the cervix also shows no abnormality...'

He's showing off, I thought, and just as I thought he was about to spoil everything, I noticed it. At first I had to blink hard to make sure what I was looking at was a reality, but unfortunately for Neil, it was. The narrow part of his red and green tartan tie had somehow found its way into her vagina underneath the speculum. Neil couldn't see it, but we could. I nudged Paul and nodded towards the perineum. Desperately, we both tried to stifle giggles. Mr Benson must have sensed this, and realising something was amiss, moved closer to Neil.

When I'd been at grammar school, from the age of about thirteen, I'd developed a way of trying to stop myself laughing when being told off by certain teachers. I'd fold my arms and nip myself as hard as I could on the sides of my chest. The pain would stop me from laughing. Usually. One night back then I'd taken off my shirt and my mam asked me what all the little bruises were. She just shook her head when I told her. I was nipping myself again but this time it wasn't working.

An understanding smile crept across Mr Benson's face. He apologised to the patient and explained Neil's unfortunate mistake before starting to laugh too. So did the patient. Neil's face was glowing red, and although I did feel sorry for him and sympathised, that wasn't going to stop Paul and I telling the rest of our group that night in the pub.

After this attachment were a few weeks in Emergency Medicine again, then Psychiatry for eight weeks. Although I had no interest in this as a career, I found it interesting, but at times it could also be frightening. At one lunchtime meeting our group was introduced to a man who was around forty-five and well dressed. He looked healthy and physically, he was. But sadly, that didn't matter to him and he may as well have had severe COPD and been in a wheelchair, unable to walk.

The psychiatrist began by asking him his name and age, and where he lived. No problem with this. But then as the questions became ever so slightly more involved, the diagnosis became clear to us even though we knew nothing at all about psychiatric illness. Simple arithmetic was beyond him and it was pitiful to see him struggle with the answers.

'Count back from thirty in threes, so twenty-seven, twenty-four and so on,' was met with a blank expression.

'Errr...' A long pause then, 'Errr...' then silence.

He was visibly uncomfortable, shuffling in his seat, embarrassed.

'What kind of shop might you buy bread or cakes in?'

Again, more awkward shifting, but silence, looking at the ground, rubbing his forehead now. After he left, we were told he had severe dementia of recent onset and was in care as he was unable to look after himself. We were told that the prognosis for this was awful and he would continue to deteriorate at a rapid rate. He would leave taps running and had caused the house to flood. He would leave the gas cooker rings burning and this had once caused a fire. It was so sad but also scary to us – he'd been perfectly normal until a couple of years earlier. Now there was no hope, he'd steadily deteriorate and need full-time care.

There were enjoyable experiences during this time too. One of the best days in the whole of medical school training for me was spent at Rainhill and Park Lane Hospitals on the outskirts of Liverpool. These housed dangerous psychiatric patients in the same way as the better-known Broadmoor. We'd spent the morning in Rainhill, then afterwards had gone to Park Lane Hospital in Maghull, now Ashworth Hospital. We were searched and had to go through several steel doors before entering one of the units, which contained around thirty men.

I noticed one, very slight with slicked back greying hair. He was immaculately dressed and ironing shirts. The prison officer pointed him out and nodded in his direction. 'That man is an infamous poisoner,' he explained. Apparently he'd experimented on his workmates, slowly poisoning them. He'd killed two and almost murdered two more. 'I know who he is,' I said. 'Graham Young.'

My three colleagues smiled. They were aware of my interest in crime and in particular, murder. They knew I'd miss the occasional day of medical school training to sit in the Crown Court, at that time in St George's Hall on Lime Street, whenever there was an interesting case being heard. I was always reading books about true crime and any years later, as a consultant on the Isle of Man, I'd write a true crime book, *Manx Murders*. Throughout my consultant career I'd follow interesting murder cases, often at the Old Bailey in London. The prison officer was amazed that I seemed to know as much about Young's crimes as he did.

I'd read about the case in a book just a few years earlier but I'd also closely followed the trial in the newspaper in 1972, when I was fifteen. When Graham Young had been about fourteen he'd started to poison his own family, killing his stepmother. He was sent to Broadmoor for a minimum of fifteen years but was released after nine. His fascination had continued though, and he'd read extensively about poisons while incarcerated, even poisoning staff and other inmates. Almost immediately after release he'd started to poison his workmates which had resulted in a life sentence. He died in prison in 1990, aged forty-two.

The end of the psychiatry attachment marked the end of year four. Each year the amount of holidays had decreased steadily. In year one there were three ten-week terms. In the final year though there would only be two weeks of holiday allowed during the whole year. Things were hotting up. Four years completed, only one to go.

The first term of year five was to be a repeat of medicine for six weeks at Broadgreen Hospital, then it was six weeks of surgery at Southport, which took us up to Christmas 1981. After the Christmas break we were on the home straight. 1982 and I'd decided, as I did at the end of my first year in a hall of residence, that I needed to move away from my friends to have the peace and quiet I needed to study. Most of my friends shared a house so the temptation to go out to the pubs was always there for them. I moved to a small flat in Crosby, between Liverpool and Southport.

Finals were due to start in May and would last about four weeks. Before that we had a couple of weeks each in ENT (Ear Nose and Throat) and ophthalmology (eyes) at St Paul's Hospital in Liverpool. Then it was two weeks in anaesthesia, first at the Royal then the Women's Hospital.

Of all the specialties, this was the one that most interested me. As an anaesthetist it seemed to me that you were your own boss. It was a fascinating specialty, as much an art as a science. There were no letters to dictate, no boring ward rounds and even more tedious clinics to attend. After a busy day working on a gynaecology list with Chris Wells, a consultant anaesthetist at the Women's Hospital, he told me he felt I should seriously think about a career as an anaesthetist. He seemed to think I had some kind of aptitude for the specialty.

It all seemed somehow more relaxed now. We were slowly winding down with clinical work, but the same couldn't be said for studying. There was plenty of that to do in preparation for our finals which were due to start in May and would take place over a four-week period.

It was during this time that I started thinking about where I would go after I had completed my degree. My favourite uncle and my dad's best friend Doug, the husband of my dad's older sister Vi, had suffered a heart attack while on holiday in the Isle of Man in October 1978. At that time I couldn't have pointed out the Isle of Man on a map, but a fellow medical student, Scott Fraser, was Manx. His mother was a GP on the island and I'd spoken to him a few times and had learnt a little about the TT motorcycle races, so I had a vague vision of the place.

After my uncle's heart attack, I met him at the Pier Head in Liverpool. A nurse had accompanied him on the ferry back to Liverpool and handed him over to my Auntie Vi and my cousins, Kathryn and Margaret, who had driven down to pick him up. They'd left the island and gone home for a week while he'd been kept in hospital. We'd had a meal together in the Berni Inn at the Pier Head, then they had driven him home to Stanley while I caught the ferry across the Mersey and made my own way home to my tiny bedsit in Birkenhead.

Now, for some reason I've never really understood, I'd started to think about this and so, one night, in February 1982, I rang him to ask him his opinion of the island. He said the island was beautiful, the staff in the hospital had been lovely, and he couldn't fault the care he'd received there.

That was good enough for me. I decided I would apply there to do my house officer jobs and wrote to the hospital management at Noble's Hospital. Without an interview, I was accepted to start work in July. My friends couldn't understand why I wanted to go there. Many of them were hoping to go to the Royal, Broadgreen, Walton or Arrowe Park. Some of them felt it was a bad career move but I didn't care.

I hated the teaching hospitals in the middle of town, always busy, with little car parking and didn't like the egos of some of the consultants who worked in them. I looked forward to a quieter life, the beaches close by, and country walks just minutes from the hospital. If my Uncle Doug liked it, I knew I would too.

May finally arrived, and finals came and went. There'd been written papers then clinicals in surgery, medicine, paediatrics and obstetrics. I felt reasonably confident, but nagging doubts would still creep in now and then. As usual, I was sitting at the bar of the King's Arms near the Royal on that Thursday evening in mid-May 1982. I was waiting for the results to be posted on typed sheets of paper at seven o'clock. These would be attached to the inside of a window in the Duncan building, adjacent to the Royal, as was the tradition.

The atmosphere in the packed pub was incredible, the tension slowly building towards the moment we'd all find out whether we'd passed or failed. Tommy, the owner, was dressed in his best suit and had put some snacks on the bar. He'd been part of our lives for three years and was clearly enjoying being part of our big night. He was a lovely man and seemed to think of us as 'his boys,' and wanted the night to be a special one we'd never forget. At around 6.50 pm others started to leave the bar and head off to get their results. Neil got up to go, but I didn't.

'I'm not going. Can you get my result for me?' I asked. I ordered another pint of lager as he set off with a few others. If you asked me why I didn't go with him, I'd struggle to put into words the true reason because I don't really know it and never will. It might be the same reason I don't feel comfortable carrying a briefcase. An inherent modesty maybe? An arguable fault to some, but something that's always been out of my control.

In May 1944 my dad, then aged nineteen, had pulled dead bodies out the sea during Exercise Tiger, after a thousand or so young Americans were torpedoed by German E-boats off Slapton Sands in Devon. This was six weeks before D-Day and they'd died during rehearsals for the invasion. He would often talk about it and just before he died seventy years later, he had become almost obsessed with finding out as much as he could about this incident. He always felt bad about it and felt strongly the British and US

Governments had let those men and their families down. He was also there on D-Day itself, off Omaha Beach on a minesweeper as a gunner. I felt that becoming a doctor was nothing compared to the sacrifices he and my mother's older brother had made.

Harry had flown to Normandy in a Glider in the early hours of June 6th 1944 so would possibly have flown over my dad's minesweeper that night as they all patiently waited in the Channel with five thousand other ships and boats for the invasion to begin. Harry never came home and will forever be in Benouville Cemetery, having died on D-Day at the age of twenty-five.

In 2004, years after that long wait in the bar to hear whether I'd qualified as a doctor, on the 60th anniversary of D-Day, I travelled to Normandy with my mam and dad and a group of veterans. I spent a week there, my first and only time in France. Every day we set off in the coach, visiting Omaha Beach, Caen, Pegasus Bridge and various British Commonwealth military cemeteries. It was fascinating to hear the stories of some of the veterans. Billy Ness from Newcastle was only nineteen and in the 12th Battalion the Parachute Regiment when he jumped out of a plane just after midnight on D-Day. During the battle he'd been shot twice. I asked him if he'd been scared. 'We didn't give a monkey's' he said, 'I was more scared of my mother. She didn't know I was there, if she'd known she'd have killed me'.

In one of the cemeteries I walked past the graves with him. He stopped at one and shook his head. 'He was one of my best mates. When you look at it you just see a headstone. When I look I see him when he was eighteen, laughing his head off, he'll always be eighteen to me. I often think about him, and why he died and I'm still here sixty years later.' Billy died in May 2021 in Newcastle, as I finished writing this book. It was an honour to have met him.

One day we went to see Harry's grave. As we stood there silently one of our group turned away and seemed to be fiddling with something in his hands as my mam laid a wreath she'd brought with her. The other ex-soldiers and my dad suddenly stood to attention as the bugle notes of *Last Post* wailed on his tape recorder. I glanced at my mam. She looked so small and I could see in her face the pain of the loss she'd suffered for all those years. I fought back tears. It was a special moment in my life, and as we got back on the coach I thanked the man with the tape recorder. 'We always do that when someone has a relative buried there,' he'd said. To me my father and uncle were brave and inspiring. Maybe this was why I found it difficult to accept that just reading books and studying, no matter how hard it might seem to me, and no matter for how long, was not something to overly celebrate.

Half an hour later and Neil was back. By then the pub was packed and the noise deafening. 'Congratulations, Doctor!' he said delightedly, and offered his hand. It is almost impossible to describe how I felt in the following few seconds. I've often compared it to the feeling of my head being about to explode. A wild combination of exhilaration and relief, excitement and pride all rolled into one swirling energy inside my head. Over-dramatic perhaps, but accurate. It was an incredible feeling, the build-up of actually getting into medical school in the first place, the ups and downs along the way. The successes and exam failures. The nightmare scenario of potentially hurting the young girl during the dreaded vaginal speculum examination in the final exam and failing because of that. The five years of study alongside all the drinking and fun. I'd made it.

I asked Neil about the rest of my little group. They'd all passed, including Chas. Euphoric, yet composed, I fought my way through the crowded bar, shaking hands, patting people on the back, and kissing. I reached the payphone and rang my mam to let her know I'd passed. She must have wondered if that day would ever come. Each time I'd arrived at Durham station at the end of a term, fifteen times in all over the five years, I'd been met by my dad patiently waiting for me on the platform. Always standing in the same spot, as if he'd never left it since ten or twelve weeks before when I'd left to head back to Liverpool. I'd always be under the 'affluence of incahol,' due to drinking during the train journey all the way from Liverpool.

On the way home from the station, my dad and I would stop off for a couple of drinks in a pub in Durham, usually the Garden House. Once home, we'd have something to eat then a few more pints in the Red Lion, a mile from home. The night before I left home to head back to Liverpool, we would have another drinking session, so when my mam and dad dropped me off at the station in Durham, I'd typically have a bit of a hangover. She must have often wondered how I'd ever qualify as a doctor. I wondered too. Or qualify for anything, in fact. Now, looking back, I feel bad that she must have worried constantly.

I was still on the phone to her when a friend, Paul Green, walked into the overflowing pub. I'd already heard he'd failed everything – medicine, surgery and obstetrics and gynaecology. He was almost in tears and I asked the barman to give him a double whiskey. I watched from the other end of the bar as he picked up the drink, but then saw his hands were shaking uncontrollably. He dropped it and it smashed on the floor. I went over and chatted with him before he left for an uncertain future.

Chas walked in with his dad who'd travelled from Hull. The bar was so full I couldn't get near him and I knew he'd just come from the station and wouldn't yet know if he'd passed. He'd told me after his last viva the examiners had said he was on very thin ice and needed to do well or he'd fail, so he knew it could go either way. His dad sat down and Chas went to the bar. Neil went over and must have told him he'd passed everything. I watched closely. The news was sinking in. Fumbling in his pocket for money, Chas's hand was shaking. He rubbed his eyes then held his face in his hands. He was crying.

It was an emotional night for everyone and one I'll never forget. We spent the rest of the night celebrating in a nightclub and the following night Euan, Paul, Chas and I caught the midnight train to London from Lime Street Station for a few days of drinking and relaxing. While I was there though I couldn't sleep at all and on the Sunday morning I decided I was going home. I was exhausted from lack of sleep.

After saying goodbye to the others at King's Cross Station, I caught the train up to Durham. I got talking to a man in the seat opposite and we had a few cans of lager together. I felt the tension caused by the buzz of the last few days slowly disappear.

That night we all celebrated in the Red Lion and later I slept for the first time since the results had come out. It was a great feeling. I then had four lazy weeks at home before I was due to start work in the Isle of Man. I'd spend every lunchtime in the local pub, chatting and playing space invaders with an old school-mate, without a care in the world. One afternoon though I was walking home and my mam was talking to a neighbour outside her house.

'I was just telling Elaine we should be at your graduation in Liverpool now. It's today.'

Again, I can't explain why, but I'd decided I wasn't going. It's another great regret I have. The truth is I was selfish and should have gone if only for my mam. To try and redeem myself I promised her if I ever passed a postgraduate degree I'd take them both to that. Five years later they came to London with us where I was presented with my MRCP degree at the Royal College of Physicians near Regent's Park. Years later, when I went to our daughter Katie's graduation in Canterbury Cathedral, I realised how much my mam would have enjoyed my own.

As the days passed in Sacriston, it gradually dawned on me that the moment I had to actually start work as a junior doctor was fast approaching. Although looking forward to at last getting stuck in, there was a distinct feeling of trepidation too.

Would I be okay, and able to cope with whatever challenges I had to face, like talking to dying patients and their relatives? Would I manage to stay calm during life-or-death situations like cardiac arrests or major trauma? Would I do a good enough job throughout the year so I'd be signed off by my consultant at the end and able to move on to the next step, an SHO job? Would I be able to walk the tightrope of being humble when that was required, but also, at other times, stand my ground and be tough enough to stand up for what I believed was right?

That day arrived, Monday July 26th, 1982. Minutes away from nine o'clock, I waited anxiously on ward five for the arrival of Mr Lee, the consultant surgeon, and his ward round. I would be working under him for the next three months. I was hoping I'd be good enough.

CHAPTER 6

Noble's

Monday July 26th 1982 and at last the day had come when I'd start work as a house officer at Noble's Hospital. I'd flown from Carlisle airport to the Isle of Man two days earlier. It was a tiny plane with an elderly lady as the only other passenger. My luggage consisted of a second-hand TV with a rope that my dad had tied around it as a handle and a small holdall. It was my first time on the island.

After medical school the next step for every newly qualified doctor was to spend a year in a pre-registration post, more commonly known as a house job. Having my name on the provisional GMC register allowed me to be able to work in an approved training post for a year and this would consist of six months each in medicine and surgery. Only if my consultants were satisfied with my performance during that year could I be signed off. My name would then appear on the full register.

Noble's was a 240 bedded District General Hospital serving a population of around 75,000. Half of my first six months were to be spent in general surgery, followed by six weeks in orthopaedics. Six weeks in obstetrics and gynaecology would follow.

The next six months would be in medicine when I would learn more about such conditions as diabetes, asthma, ischaemic heart disease and chronic lung disease. Six weeks would be spent in paediatrics.

Five other house officers shared the nights and weekends on call with me. We'd attend ward rounds, following the consultant, registrar and SHO like ducklings faithfully trailing behind their mother towards water. My job was essentially to write a summary of the consultant's findings and decisions in the case notes, making a note of any instructions, writing up drugs and generally carrying out any directions left by the consultant or registrar. I'd take blood samples and organise various investigations such as X-rays and scans.

A good relationship with nursing staff made the whole process much easier as they would usually recognise our inexperience and be willing to help us in any way they could. I would now say, looking back, I learnt as much about caring for patients from nurses as I did from other doctors.

We would have to ensure the operating list was given to the typist in theatre who would check the relevant wards had a copy, before letting the X-ray department know if the surgeon would need them to assist during routine operating lists, in order that they could allocate a radiographer to theatre. When on call we'd be contacted by GPs about patients who required admission to hospital and it was down to us to arrange where each patient would go, to a ward or to A&E. A house officer would see them first and decide who needed to be contacted for advice on further management.

Another route into the hospital for a patient was via the A&E department. It was again our responsibility to assess the patient there by taking a history, carrying out an examination and ordering relevant investigations before formulating a diagnosis, if this was possible. In reality, it would usually be a differential diagnosis because the precise one might not be known until results of blood tests and other investigations were back or it might be only revealed at the time of surgery.

After we'd seen the patient, we would usually have to inform the SHO, next in rank to us, what we had discovered and he might also check our findings.

If surgery was planned a consent form had to be completed. A discussion would take place involving a description of the proposed operation, the potential complications that could follow and the possibility of further surgery if unanticipated findings indicated this was necessary.

For example, if appendicitis was suspected in a girl and at surgery the actual problem was found to be a twisted ovary, the ovary might have to be removed. If there was felt to be a high likelihood of any part of the bowel being removed, a warning would be given that a stoma might be required. This might be needed if there was a significant risk that the joined bowel might not heal and potentially fall apart causing a bowel leak and peritonitis, which could carry a very high mortality rate. The contents of the bowel would pass into a stoma bag rather than via the rectum and anus.

But for me, the best part of my surgery attachment was assisting in the operating theatre, seeing the pathology which had caused the patient's symptoms and physical signs. Mr Lee was renowned for his lengthy operating lists, due to being one of only two consultant surgeons in the hospital at that time, and on several occasions I would be assisting him until the list finished. One Friday evening, I had made arrangements to meet up with some of my colleagues in one of the local pubs at 7 o'clock, however, the last case of the day took around six hours and only finished at 9.30pm. When I eventually joined them around 10pm, they weren't too surprised, but I wasn't happy. The following morning at 9am, as with every Saturday morning for that 12-week attachment, I was expected to join him on his ward round even if I wasn't on call. Nowadays, due to the implementation of the European Working Time Directive, requiring the working week to be an average of 48 hours, this sort of thing simply wouldn't happen. As a junior doctor and even as a registrar and senior registrar, I would regularly be expected to be available to work for around 70-80 hours a week.

Slowly, almost imperceptibly, we began to gain experience and confidence in diagnosing and treating surgical conditions such as appendicitis, bowel obstruction, pancreatitis, gastric and duodenal ulcers, bowel and rectal cancer and cholecystitis (inflammation of the gallbladder).

The hospital in the Isle of Man was probably at that time unique in one respect.

As house officers, the most inexperienced doctors in the hospital, we were required to also work as A&E doctors. There were no consultants in this specialty at that time, and only two regular doctors working there. We would cover this department on nights and weekends when they weren't able to do so and were paid extra for this work. Most of the others didn't enjoy or feel comfortable with this work and I would often do their shifts.

I feel it would be almost certainly correct to say that none of the one hundred and forty or so of my fellow ex-students would be working in any UK hospital unsupervised in an A&E department. We did, of course, have back up, from the SHO and registrar in medicine and surgery, but we were the ones seeing the patients first, then deciding initial management and who to refer to for further advice and management. It was terrifying at times but looking back it was a fantastic way of gaining experience as a very junior doctor. The nurses were well aware of our inexperience and helped and supported us.

During my time as a house officer in surgery I became interested in learning more about anaesthetics, which I'd enjoyed during my two-week attachment as a medical student. I'd also liked ophthalmology, or eye surgery, as a student. On my first day at Noble's I tracked down the eye surgeon, Mr Travers. I told him I was interested in his own specialty and was trying to decide between a career in that or anaesthetics. He'd said if I wanted to I was welcome to spend time with him in the clinic and theatre. I never did. I soon became more interested in what the anaesthetist was doing than the surgery itself.

I'd go into the anaesthetic room to watch the anaesthetist who worked with Mr Lee, Dougie Leece, put his patients to sleep. He was a Manxman who had trained in Manchester then worked in Blackpool before starting at Noble's in the early seventies. He was a real character with an infectious laugh. Often the patient would be terrified and he had his own way of putting them at ease.

He'd kneel on the floor, gently tap the back of the patient's hand to help 'get the veins up' and say,

'I'm just going to plunge six inches of stainless steel into the back of your hand, nothing to worry about.'

Then he'd glance at the patient and burst into laughter.

It never failed and the patient and the nurse would laugh too.

He'd let me intubate the patient and then I'd go into the theatre, wash my hands then assist the surgeon with the operation. If I wasn't needed to scrub up and assist during surgery I'd sit next to Dougie and ask him questions about being an anaesthetist and training in the specialty. To me it was fascinating, seeing the patient wake up within minutes of being anaesthetised. I'd always known that surgery was not for me but I wanted a specialty where I could use my hands to intubate the airway, put in IV lines, draw up and inject drugs, fiddle with ventilators in the Intensive Care Unit (ICU). I was far more interested in anaesthesia than surgery. By the end of my three months of surgery I'd decided that might be my future and Dougie would be part of the interview committee for a consultant post at Noble's, seven years later.

The hospital consultants by then knew I was very keen to return to Noble's. When a consultant job came up I applied, although I knew I was a bit short on experience as a senior registrar. Three others were short-listed too, they were all already consultants and one had been working on the island for a year or so as a locum. After the interviews ended, we were all told that no one had been appointed. They'd decided they were going to re-advertise the post in six months or so. I knew what that meant. The Royal College of Anaesthetists' representative on the interview committee had, as I expected, said he couldn't support my

If In Doubt

appointment as I needed another six months of training. Although the other three were all appointable, Dougie and the consultant surgeon from the hospital said they wanted me to get the job and it was decided to re-advertise later. It was the first time I'd been unsuccessful in an interview. Six months later I was appointed.

I owe a lot to Dougie. He was a great anaesthetist and a lovely man. I felt proud when a few of the experienced recovery nurses who'd worked with him for many years would tell me he thought of me as his protégé.

Dougie told me that working as an anaesthetist at Noble's was a great job with lots of variety - so long as everything went well. On a small island however, with only a few anaesthetists, any serious mistake would be big news in the media and any reputation you might have built up could quickly disappear. He said he never allowed himself to forget that.

Towards the end of my year at Noble's, in 1983, I was working in the A&E department, now known as the ED (Emergency Department – throughout this book I use these terms interchangeably). Something was about to happen which was to have a profound impact on me and I still think of it now and then even today.

That would become the weekend I decided I wanted to be an anaesthetist.

The nurses on duty that day knew that I had no idea how to deal with many of the patients and they were very supportive. If I was really struggling and they felt they couldn't help me, they would suggest that I contact the on-call registrar in medicine or surgery and sometimes psychiatry for advice, so there was always that reassuring back-up if it was needed. They'd have seen the patient before I did so they had an idea of what might be wrong with them.

At around 3pm a nurse told me they'd had a call from an ambulance to let the A&E staff know that a young lady, aged twenty, was being brought in having collapsed at a nearby swimming pool. She'd suddenly felt unwell while swimming in the pool and had become breathless and had felt faint. She'd clambered out and lay on the poolside.

My initial thought was that this would not be a serious admission to A&E, perhaps a simple fainting episode. As I awaited her arrival, I looked at a couple of other patients who were already occupying beds, one with a nasty wrist fracture sustained playing football. It was a compound fracture, a jagged piece of bone had pierced the skin and required urgent debridement, cleaning of the wound and intravenous antibiotics. The main concern with this type of injury is osteomyelitis, infection in the bone itself, which can be very difficult to treat. An elderly man had fallen and fractured his hip. It was clear both would require surgery to fix their broken bones and I rang the orthopod on call to let him know there were two customers for him.

The rest of the department was quiet but that was about to change.

About half an hour later, I was talking to the orthopaedic SHO and looking at the X-ray of the hip fracture illuminated on the viewing box. A nurse told me the lady from the pool, Sally, had just been brought in and didn't look too good to her. The fear and concern in her voice triggered my adrenaline; I needed to see her immediately.

We walked hurriedly to the far cubicle and she pulled back the pastel-blue curtain like a magician in a magic show to reveal the surprise hidden behind it to an unsuspecting audience. Me. Even with my lack of experience it was clear that she was in serious trouble. This was not at all what I'd been expecting and I had to suppress a feeling of fear. I'd do this many times during my career. It always seemed to have the same effect on me.

It went a bit like this: I'd subconsciously start to swallow several times immediately and I'd lick my lips – my mouth would seem to instantly dry up. It would be almost like an out of body experience: I'd look down on myself asking, 'What do I look like to anyone around me, watching me?'

If In Doubt

Would I look calm and in control? If things went badly would they criticize me for not doing a good job? If it went well, might they pat me on the back and say 'Well done'?

It sounds ridiculous but I have always done that when a serious situation occurs, whether it be in the operating theatre, ED, obstetric unit, ICU or wherever. The sudden surge of adrenaline always had these effects on me and there was absolutely nothing I could do about it. I have always tried to remain in control of myself in difficult situations. Stay calm, never shout or become angry. Once control is lost vital correct decision-making goes straight out of the window. If that happens it becomes impossible to give the best care you can.

Sally was very pretty and slim with long blond hair. She was clearly frightened, sitting bolt up-right on the trolley and leaning forward slightly, in a position I'd see hundreds of times later during my career, as the patient found the best way to help their laboured breathing. Anything to make it feel a little bit easier.

She was breathing so fast she was unable to speak in a full sentence, an indication of the seriousness of her condition. I could see through the transparent plastic oxygen mask that her lips were tinged with a faint bluish colour, another very worrying sign. This blue discolouration, or cyanosis, indicates a problem when the patient is breathing air, which contains 21% oxygen. If they are cyanosed while they are receiving a very high concentration of oxygen it is even more serious. It means that the patient's life is in grave danger.

Beads of sweat had formed on her forehead in the creases that were there because of the effort of breathing and the anxiety and fear she was feeling. I often wondered how many times these masks had only served to mask the truth. Over the next thirty-eight years, I'd see it over and over again.

If a patient looks pink, surely they must be ok? Wrong.

If In Doubt

If they are not breathing added oxygen via a facemask and look pink, it's a reassuring sign. A pulse oximeter probe on a finger indicating there is an adequate level of oxygen in the blood is another positive signal. At that time pulse oximeters had not been invented, today they are used routinely and give an indication of the amount of oxygen carried in the blood. Oxygen is essential for life itself and without it a person will die within minutes.

In a situation where there is complete loss of the airway, no air can enter the lungs and pass through them into the blood. Death will occur from hypoxia, or lack of oxygen, within minutes unless the airway is reopened and oxygen passes through it into the lungs. Oxygen is usually given to any ill patient, whether they need it or not, but it has another potentially dangerous side to it.

On the one hand it is life-saving, on the other it can lull the unsuspecting or inexperienced nurse or doctor into a dangerous false sense of security and by keeping the patient pink and oximeter reading normal the seriousness of the illness might not be appreciated. If the oxygen hadn't been given, cyanosis would have been seen and the low oxygen reading on the oximeter would have left no one, however inexperienced or unwary, in any doubt that the patient's life was in imminent danger.

Her hands felt cool and clammy, damp with sweat, with a raised respiratory rate of around thirty breaths per minute. Very fast.

I was immediately worried.

She said she'd had a cold but hadn't felt particularly ill with it. There'd been a slight dry cough and nasal discharge for the previous few days. She'd been swimming, but had felt a little dizzy, climbed out of the pool then felt faint. She'd lain down on the poolside and suddenly felt breathless. We don't even think about breathing normally. It just happens. The awareness of it being difficult is termed 'dyspnoea.' She hadn't experienced any chest pain.

Something was very wrong here. I realised immediately I needed help and asked a nurse to call the on-call registrar in medicine urgently.

A normally fit, healthy young lady had in a very short space of time developed shortness of breath apparently without warning. There was no history of asthma and no recent trauma which might have led to a pneumothorax. In this condition, a leak develops in the lining of the lung, the pleura. Air that would normally stay within the lung passes into the space around it via the hole in the pleura and gradually accumulates in this pleural cavity and causes the lung to collapse as the pressure around it increases. It can occur spontaneously or following trauma, often with associated rib fractures. That was a possible cause in the list of differential diagnoses.

I quickly obtained a history and examined her. I listened to her chest and heard crackles on inspiration at the lung bases. Normally on auscultation, or listening with a stethoscope to the sound of air going in and out, a kind of whooshing sound is heard but no added sounds.

Crackles might indicate heart failure. If she'd lost consciousness in the pool some water could have flowed into her lungs but she'd been fully conscious throughout so there was no question of drowning as a differential diagnosis.

I asked the nurse if she could organise a portable chest X-ray and filled in the request form for that. Although not really expecting to see any abnormality on it, I also asked for an ECG, or electrocardiogram, to look for heart abnormalities. Scanning over this quickly it was immediately apparent that the situation was critical.

On a normal ECG the electrical activity of the heart on the trace is regular, with a pulse rate of around seventy beats per minute. The spikes (complexes) are usually quite narrow and there are other waveforms, which to anyone familiar with looking at ECGs are easily seen to be normal or abnormal.

If In Doubt

This one was far from normal, displaying a rate of 120 beats per minute. The QRS complexes were wide and there were ectopics - extra beats. Having contacted the medical registrar and told him that although I had no idea what was wrong with this young lady, I was now even more worried about her and felt she may be best monitored in the CCU, or Coronary Care Unit. Another doctor soon appeared and agreed that the CCU was the appropriate place for her to be closely monitored.

The chest X-ray was brought to A&E by the radiographer. She appeared to be very concerned about the image she'd processed. She placed it on the viewing box and I saw that there was pulmonary congestion, a generalised excess of fluid in the lungs with a white-out of both lungs indicating possible heart failure. On a chest X-ray air appears black, fluid white.

The lungs, instead of being filled with air, were full of fluid. Although rare, I wondered if this could be viral myocarditis, a rare condition where there is inflammation of the cardiac muscle caused by a viral infection.

She was quickly transferred from A&E to the CCU just across the corridor and I felt a sense of relief to be getting back to my A&E duties. For the next few hours, I treated a few more patients with more minor injuries from Saturday afternoon sports; a broken ankle, broken fingers from a motocross crash and one patient with an eye injury that fortunately didn't require treatment.

My shift in A&E ended at eight o'clock and instinctively I went back to the CCU on my way back to my room, which was in the hospital, to check on her. I was told she'd just been moved into the adjoining ICU and I wandered into the side room there.

Breathing even faster now, she was requiring an even higher percentage of oxygen.

The pulmonary congestion, fluid on the lungs, was clearly worsening. A nurse whispered that her latest chest

X-ray had looked much worse than the first one. Her anxious parents sat on either side of the bed.

I could see she was now finding it more difficult to speak. A consultant anaesthetist walked into the room and nodded to me, at the same time glancing at the name badge pinned to the breast pocket of my white coat. I'd never seen him before. He'd been called in from home by the consultant physician on call as it was felt that the girl's condition was deteriorating rapidly and she might soon need to be put onto a ventilator.

I went to my room and lay on the bed watching TV for an hour or so before heading out to join the others for a few drinks. I found myself going over the events in ED during the evening. It was midnight by the time I got back to the hospital and on my way to my room I felt drawn back towards the ICU. Looking back now, as I write this, thirty-eight years later, I realise it was the start of a pattern.

With some patients I have become involved to the extent that I felt the need to constantly see them and watch their progress – or deterioration – and become involved in their ongoing care. While I have tried to keep away when not on call and therefore technically not responsible for any decision-making, I've at times found it difficult. I think my colleagues could see I was only doing it because I wanted the best for the patient and it almost never caused a problem. I was always conscious that I couldn't overstep the mark and interfere with treatment when it wasn't my place to do so. The GMC, the doctor's regulating body, would take a dim view of that.

Her condition had by now deteriorated even further while I'd been out and she'd been anaesthetised and intubated. A tracheal tube had been inserted so that she could be attached to the ventilator because she couldn't breathe on her own any longer. The ventilator was delivering 70% oxygen.

Throughout my career as an anaesthetist when looking after ICU patients on ventilators this is one of the first things

I always ask about or look at. I must have asked that question many thousands of times.

If a patient is requiring only 30% oxygen, not much more than the 21% present in air, their respiratory function is probably not too bad and they might be considered suitable for being weaned, or taken off the ventilator. On the other hand, if say 85% inspired oxygen was needed to ensure that enough of it entered the blood, it would be clear that there was no prospect of the patient being able to breathe on their own and there was a serious problem in the lungs.

Common causes for this are pneumonia, heart failure, lung contusion (bruising of the lungs caused by trauma to the chest) and ARDS (Adult Respiratory Distress Syndrome).

ARDS occurs when the human body mounts a response to an underlying illness or severe infection such as peritonitis, pancreatitis, massive blood loss and major trauma or a serious burn injury. The release of various chemicals from cells in the body appear to somehow attack the lungs and fluid and cells can leak into the tissues there and cause worsening respiratory function and a typical X-ray appearance, with patchy shadowing throughout both lungs. There is no real treatment for this apart from supportive measures and managing the underlying condition. It carries a high mortality rate which to me doesn't seem to have changed over the last thirty years or so despite changes in drug therapy.

It still wasn't clear what the diagnosis of Sally's illness was, but she was being treated for cardiac failure. I wasn't on duty the next day, Sunday. I'd move into a flat a few weeks later where I'd live for the rest of my time as a house officer when not on call. At that time, though, my room was only about fifty yards from the ICU right in the middle of the hospital. During that day I'd been in and out a few times, reading the case notes, trying to follow the chain of thought of the more senior doctors as they battled to save her. I chatted to the nurses and to Pete, the SHO in anaesthetics, about Sally's condition.

Like sentinels guarding a most precious jewel, her devastated parents had kept watch every hour of the night, and now, as they had the previous afternoon, sat motionless either side of the bed. Neither spoke but gazed despairingly at her pale face and the nasogastric tube that protruded unnaturally from her nose. A red rubber tube was taped securely to her right cheek, the tube exiting the corner of her mouth on the right side. Her eyes had been taped shut to prevent any potential for corneal damage and a central venous line with three lumens entered the right side of her neck, coursing its way into the internal jugular vein and secured with a transparent dressing, carrying fluid and the drugs that were supporting her heart and keeping her anaesthetised.

A nurse chatted to her as she injected a drug into the three-way tap attached to the line as if she was fully conscious. All ICU nurses do this and they tell parents or other patient relatives to do the same. It's odd, really. I thought it strange then and now after all these years I still do.

We all know the chance of the patient actually hearing anything we say is practically zero. The patient is anaesthetised in the same way a patient having surgery would be. We don't talk to those patients in the operating theatre. If we did, we might find ourselves being urgently referred to a psychiatrist.

Do we do it as an attempt to desperately try to keep that human bond that is an innate part of our own existence? We can't make eye contact because the eyes are taped shut and the patient can't talk because he or she is unconscious. Even if they weren't they'd still be mute because a plastic tube with an internal diameter of about seven or eight millimetres lies between the vocal cords.

But there is no physical barrier between our mouths and the patient's ears. Maybe that is the link needed to keep us both in some sort of tenuous human contact? An invisible bond of hope, maybe? I don't know, but it's something I think about even many years later. Will I 'get it' before I stop work completely, I would wonder, or is there no real answer?

There'd been discussions with other intensive care doctors in Liverpool in a desperate attempt to give Sally the best chance of life, but as I read the summary of these, it was clear that they too were at a loss to know what else could be done at that time. Their advice had been clear. Transferring her to Liverpool by air ambulance wasn't an option. Moving her would have been risky and they felt there was nothing more they could do. Press on and hope for the best was all they could offer.

Her parents were aware that she was critically ill and might die soon. I must have been in and out about four times and at nine o'clock that night I wandered in again, hoping for any sign of improvement.

I heard raised voices from outside the room even before I entered.

A few minutes earlier the level of sedative drugs must have been inadequate because she had started to cough and gag on the tracheal tube and had suddenly started to thrash around. The tracheal tube had come out. It appeared that the IV cannula in her left arm may have tissued – the tip had come out of the vein and into the surrounding tissues. Therefore the drugs keeping her asleep had gone outside the vein instead of into her blood where they would have been carried to the brain and ensured she remained in a coma. They'd given a bolus of the drug into her neck line and she was again unconscious but pink froth was now pouring out of her mouth. It was frank pulmonary oedema fluid, a sign of very severe left ventricular heart failure; it was as if her very life was rapidly leaving her body.

In fact, that is precisely what was happening.

The anaesthetist, an Asian man, who was tall, balding, vacant and silent, stood behind Sally's head. He was leaning forward, his right hand guiding a suction catheter in and out of her mouth, past the blue-coloured lips, trying to keep the airway clear.

The Sister was by now screaming at him to re-intubate her.

'Put the fucking tube back in! What are you waiting for? Here's the laryngoscope. For Christ's sake!'

She glared at him. But he just kept on with the futile suctioning, appearing to be in some sort of trance.

The pink froth poured out of her mouth as well as into the suction tube.

'Dr Gelling's on his way, he told me not to do anything until he gets here,' he mumbled, his voice almost unheard, drowned out by the noise of the suction machine and the ventilator alarms.

The nurse shook her head angrily.

'She'll be dead by the time he gets here, get the tube back in, she's not getting any oxygen at all now! For Christ's sake do something!' Still no response.

More suctioning. No one spoke.

Waiting for the inevitable.

The sucker bottle was slowly filling with the fizzy pink froth. I stood inches from him. Even as an inexperienced doctor it was clear to me that the one thing that had to be done was for the tracheal tube to be put back in immediately and oxygen needed to be squeezed into her lungs.

He must have had the same thought because he suddenly inserted the laryngoscope into her mouth to re-intubate her. As he did so, the ECG complexes widened then slowed, thirty, fourteen, no complexes.

A blank screen.

Asystole – cardiac arrest. The inevitable outcome we all knew was coming.

I stepped forward, shaking my head instinctively and started chest compressions as the anaesthetist tried desperately to force oxygen into her fluid-filled lungs through a face mask. The medical SHO and registrar were now in the room and intravenous adrenaline was injected into the neck line.

No change in the ECG, still asystole. Even I knew it was completely hopeless.

As I continued with chest compressions, the anaesthetist continued trying to re-intubate her and asked me to stop for a second so that he could visualise the vocal cords and see where the tube was to go.

'It's too late for that now, don't bother!' the sister shouted angrily.

'She's dead, there's no point carrying on, we all know it, it's too late!'

The tube slid in easily and we carried on, each with our own thoughts, no one spoke.

The pink froth now went into the breathing circuit instead of flooding from her mouth, flowing back and forth in the transparent blue plastic tube connecting the patient to the ventilator.

After a few more minutes, the medical registrar said he felt we should stop as it appeared futile. I nodded in agreement.

The anaesthetist said nothing. Neither did anyone else. He was close to tears and trembling slightly, averting his eyes as he walked out of the room. At that same moment Dr Gelling rushed past him into the room. He stopped in his tracks, taking in the scene.

Later, as I lay on my bed I went over the whole series of events since the phone call informing us she was on the way into the hospital from the swimming pool and ending in her death. She'd been so ill she would almost certainly have died anyway, but the end of the story had not been a good one.

The anaesthetist had not done his job. If I'd been the anaesthetist I would have stepped forward and calmly reinserted the tube, wouldn't I? Maybe I'd have even saved her?

I had thought about a career as an anaesthetist and now I wanted to be one.

At the subsequent coroner's inquest, it was found that the death was due to 'natural causes'. The post-mortem had not revealed any obvious underlying medical conditions that may have predisposed her to suddenly developing cardiac failure.

Three months after I'd started working at the hospital, at the end of October, we'd organised a doctors' party in the sitting room in our accommodation in the hospital where we had a small bar and would meet each night after work. One of the ICU nurses I worked with brought a friend. She was the most beautiful girl I'd ever seen. I was introduced to her; her name was Kerry and she was Manx and lived with her parents in Willaston on the outskirts of Douglas. We soon started going out together and the day after Boxing Day 1983, about ten weeks after we'd met, we flew to Liverpool on our way to Durham to stay with my parents for a week. I proposed to her that night in Liverpool and we decided the wedding would be at the end of TT Race Week, 11th of June. I reasoned if any of my medical school friends or anyone else wanted to come over for the wedding they could also see some racing before it.

Our wedding was the best day of my life.

My brother and two of my best friends from medical school had come to the island a week before the wedding and I'd managed to get them each a room in the doctors' residence in the hospital. My parents and some aunts and uncles, including Doug and Vi, and friends of the family flew over from Blackpool the day before. Some of my medical student friends from Liverpool came over on the ferry and Mr Lee and his wife also attended. The wedding itself was a perfect day.

We had a lovely week in London for our honeymoon and then I had six more weeks to work at Noble's. After this we loaded up the car and set off to Liverpool on the ferry for a month's holiday back home in Sacriston.

I was to start my training in Liverpool in anaesthetics at the Royal on September 1st 1983. I was going to be an anaesthetist.

CHAPTER 7

Hurdles

First it was O-levels and then A–levels.

Then there were the exams at the end of our preclinical part of the course after almost two years, the First MB. (Our degree was MB, ChB, Bachelor of Medicine, Bachelor of Surgery; the 'Ch' stands for Chirugie, the French word for surgery.)

Next were our finals, or Final MB. That was in two parts, the first after three years: pathology, pharmacology and microbiology. At the end of the five years was the Final MB: medicine, surgery and obstetrics and gynaecology.

Later there would be postgraduate exams in anaesthesia, the FFARCS (Fellowship of the Faculty of Anaesthetists in the Royal College of Surgeons as it was at that time). Now anaesthetists have their own Royal College so the title is FRCA (Fellow of the Royal College of Anaesthetists). This was the degree I had to pass if I wanted to become a consultant anaesthetist.

The equivalent qualification for a doctor hoping to be a consultant in Medicine, or a physician, is the MRCP (Member of the Royal College of Physicians). As I neared the end of my first year as a doctor on the Isle of Man, I decided I was going to try my best to achieve both.

Each of these postgraduate degrees was in two parts. I had to get the FFARCS as I wanted a career in anaesthesia and nothing else but that would do for me. If I could pass the MRCP too, I reasoned, it would make me a better doctor and anaesthetist. I'd know a lot more about diagnosing and treating medical conditions that many of my future patients who needed anaesthetics would have, as well as many of those who I'd look after in the ICU. Having the MRCP would hopefully make it easier for me to get registrar and senior registrar posts and eventually a consultant post.

I'd already decided that if I made it that far, I wanted to be a consultant on the Isle of Man if at all possible.

From the first day of training in anaesthesia, now back in Liverpool after my year in the Isle of Man, I was studying for the primary exams for these two degrees at the same time. I failed the anaesthetic exam in London the following February and also failed the first part of the MRCP the following month. This latter exam was a 300-question multiple choice paper and could be taken in several centres, fortunately one of these was Liverpool which saved me travelling.

In May 1984, I passed the primary FFARCS at my second attempt in Dublin, receiving the result on the same day our first daughter was born. A few months later in October 1984, just after I'd started a medical job for one year, I passed the first part of the MRCP.

That medical job was in cardiology and chest medicine at Broadgreen Hospital, now the Liverpool Heart and Chest Hospital. To be eligible to take the final part of the MRCP I needed a minimum of one year in an accredited medical post and this was it. After that year, I intended to return to anaesthetics and try to pass the final MRCP while working as an anaesthetist again.

My first year of training as an anaesthetist involved working for the various surgical specialties such as orthopaedics, general surgery, ENT (Ear, Nose and Throat), dental and ophthalmology at the nearby St Paul's Eye Hospital. In addition, we spent two months in the ICU in the Royal. We'd be on call every fourth or fifth night and weekend, initially doing everything with a registrar, but after four months or so we were allowed to anaesthetise straightforward patients on our own, with the registrar close by if we needed help.

The most important thing during my early training was gaining experience and confidence in managing the airway.

During the anaesthetic the patient would either breathe through a face mask or through a tracheal tube attached to a breathing circuit which in turn was attached to the anaesthetic machine. Anaesthetic gases would keep the patient anaesthetised. I'd hold a face mask for hours on end and my right hand would ache for the first few weeks. As the small muscles in my hand became stronger the aching stopped. From the mid-1980s, supraglottic airway devices were invented (SADs). Nowadays they are used on the vast majority of patients having a general anaesthetic. The airway is inserted after the patient is anaesthetised and this allows the anaesthetist's hands to be freed up. There is no need to hang on to a face mask as I did in those early days of training. Far fewer patients need tracheal intubation – the SAD has replaced the need for a tube in many cases.

After my first year of anaesthetic training, I started a medical job at Broadgreen, now the Liverpool Heart and Chest Hospital. This consisted of six months in a busy Coronary Care Unit (CCU), and three months each in cardiology and chest medicine. It was widely considered by most anaesthetists in Liverpool to be the best medical post available as the two main organs which concern any anaesthetist are the heart and lungs.

Central venous access is the term given to placing an intravenous cannula into the large veins in the neck or chest. This is inserted for various reasons including IV feeding, when irritant drugs need to be infused for prolonged periods of time and for monitoring pressures within these veins, and when peripheral veins don't exist and IV access is essential.

The procedure carries definite risks, some very serious, including puncture of nearby major arteries and haemorrhage from these and puncture of the pleura, the lining of the lung causing a pneumothorax and lung collapse, and the small risk of this developing into a pneumothorax or a tension pneumothorax.

With this rare condition a one-way valve effect can lead to an increase in the pressure within the chest cavity which drastically impedes the flow of blood in the large veins carrying it back to the heart, and if this pressure is not relieved with a chest drain to release the trapped air, it can be lethal.

When a permanent pacemaker is to be implanted, a needle is first inserted into the subclavian vein which lies behind the clavicle (collar bone). A flexible wire is then passed through the needle, a catheter over the wire which is then removed before the lead to the pacemaker is inserted through the catheter so its tip is positioned in the wall of the left ventricle. This is then connected to the control box which is placed so it lies under the skin beneath the clavicle.

I was allowed, under the supervision of the consultant cardiologist, to perform the subclavian puncture. This is the essential step in inserting an IV line into it and I soon gained confidence with this which would help me throughout my anaesthetic career. Anaesthetists are often called to insert central venous lines. That year provided me with a huge amount of knowledge and experience in treating disturbances in heart rhythm, arrhythmias, and the medical management of angina and cardiac failure, respiratory conditions like COPD and asthma among many other conditions, some of them very rare.

I would attend clinics and be on call at night, and lead any cardiac arrests as the SHO in coronary care, although if a more experienced registrar was there, they would take over this role, much to my relief. The hospital was the regional centre and so it was always busy.

During this year of medicine I would also regularly do locum anaesthetic jobs, usually at Arrowe Park hospital but also Warrington and Broadgreen, keeping my hand in and gaining more experience.

Although I had learnt about cardiology and chest medicine during that year, for the MRCP I needed to also be up to date with all the other sub-specialties like neurology, renal medicine, gastroenterology, oncology, endocrinology and even tropical medicine and psychiatry.

Next it was back to anaesthetics. I took up a registrar post at Arrowe Park Hospital on the Wirral. I was learning how to anaesthetise children for the first time and this was my first experience of obstetric anaesthesia. I learnt how to perform an epidural for labour analgesia and how to anaesthetise for caesarean section. At night and during weekends I'd be on call for either ICU or obstetrics and there would also be a SHO on-call for general anaesthesia such as trauma and surgery like appendicectomy or orthopaedics. I was actually on call there the night my wife was admitted for a ruptured ectopic pregnancy and also during the night when she went into labour with our second daughter in March 1986.

To improve my chances of success in the final MRCP I'd pester any medic I knew –and some I didn't know – into asking me questions or teaching me about various conditions.

One afternoon at Arrowe Park I was washing my hands before an epidural for a woman in labour. My bleep went off and a friend who'd recently passed his final MRCP told me that he had a quick case for me in A&E, only a hundred yards away across the car park. Drying my hands, I made an excuse that I had to do something urgently, but it would only take a few minutes, then ran over to the A&E department. He introduced me to a young man who had suddenly developed left-sided chest pain and breathlessness and watched as I examined his chest then listened as I presented my findings.

'On examination he is receiving oxygen via nasal cannulae at four litres per minute, appears short of breath but able to easily speak in sentences. Respiratory rate twenty-four per minute. Not cyanosed, trachea central, decreased expansion on the left, normal percussion note, no hyper-resonance, decreased air entry on the left with no wheeze or bronchial breathing.'

'Diagnosis?' he said.

'Left-sided pneumothorax', I replied and he smiled as I ran back and performed the epidural. I'd ring registrars in other hospitals and they'd take me on teaching rounds at night, neurology patients at Walton, cardiac patients at Broadgreen, general medical patients at Whiston and the Royal, rheumatology, anything at all that might help me learn as much as I could about medicine.

If news filtered through of anyone in Liverpool I knew passing the MRCP I'd track them down and ask if they would take me to see patients. It was no different with anaesthesia. Many years later I'd meet anaesthetists I hadn't seen since I trained with them. They'd recall I always had a book with me, reading in the coffee room in the theatre or in the ICU. I was always asking more experienced anaesthetists questions or asking them to question me. It was a way for me to learn where my weaknesses were. If I was asked a question and didn't know the answer I'd go off and learn more.

I'd heard the two-week course at Whipps Cross hospital in London was the best one for those hoping to pass the final MRCP, so off I went. I stayed with my brother-in-law Dursley in a flat in Covent Garden and travelled by train each day to the hospital. It was exhausting but I was determined to learn as much as I could to improve my chances of passing.

The final MRCP was held every four months in Glasgow, Edinburgh and London. Someone told me it might be a little easier in Glasgow. I doubted that there was really any truth in this as the same examiners rotated through all three centres. A candidate was allowed a total of six attempts only. I'd decided I'd sit the exam every four months until I either passed it or failed all six.

The first one was in Glasgow. To start, there were written papers, then I had to wait a few weeks before hearing if I was through to the clinical part. I got through and went back again to Glasgow by train from Liverpool for the clinical part. After I'd been to Monklands Hospital in Airdrie I'd caught the train back to Glasgow. I failed and rang my wife on a payphone in Glasgow Central Hotel in the train station, where I had a room.

I'd walked up to the Royal College of Surgeons in Glasgow to get my result. I was amazed to see others, men, hugging each other outside, crying. I thought it was pathetic. Maybe that was their sixth and last attempt, I wondered, but whatever the reason, it still looked bad to me. I always felt that whatever happened you still had to put everything into perspective. If you weren't good enough, face it. There seemed to be little point crying about it. You'd still failed and nothing was going to change that.

Four months later, I was back in Glasgow again for my second attempt. This time I went to Inverclyde Hospital in Greenock. I was staying at the same hotel. I suddenly had a déjà vu moment as I was dialling the same number on the same phone to again tell my wife that I'd been unsuccessful. Four trips to Glasgow and nothing to show for it. Back to square one, I had four chances left. Now, with our second baby arriving in a few weeks, I knew it would become more difficult to study at home.

Four months on and I was in London this time. I'd again passed the written part and was back for the clinical part, this time at Edgware General Hospital. As before it consisted of a long case, where I had thirty minutes to take a history and examine a patient, before being grilled by two examiners and this time it went well. The patient had multiple sclerosis and I felt I'd done reasonably well in answering their questions. I was reasonably happy so far.

Next came probably the most important part, the short cases. The idea was that during a half hour period, two examiners took you to see a series of patients, six or seven on average. I was introduced to a young lady of about twenty and I was asked to examine the retina of both eyes with an ophthalmoscope. The retina is the only part of the body where the capillaries (small blood vessels) can be clearly seen, magnified by the ophthalmoscope. He handed me one and I asked her to fix her gaze at a point behind me and try to concentrate on looking at it while I looked into her eyes. The tendency is for the patient to look at the light and this causes the pupil to constrict so that very little can be seen of the retina. By fixing on a distant point the brain tells the eye to keep the pupil open allowing more of the retina to be seen.

I saw it immediately but asked her to look up, down right and left as I tried to work out how the questioning might go.

The retina is red, the capillaries can be seen crisscrossing it. The optic nerve enters the back of the eyeball as a round pale area, the optic disc and nerve fibres which carry information back to the brain spread out through the retina but are so tiny they can't be seen with the ophthalmoscope. Before reaching the eye these fibres have a myelin sheath, a protective covering. Usually, in most people, this stops before the nerve fibres spread through the retina, but in a very small minority, it continues for a short distance along the nerves in the retina, blurring the normally sharp and clearly defined edge of the disc.

I'd never actually seen it before, but I'd seen photographs and read about it. After thirty seconds or so I thanked the patient and stood up, handed the examiner the ophthalmoscope, and waited, looking him in the eye.

'What did you find?' he enquired.

'There are no haemorrhages or exudates and the retinas appear normal, but both optic disc edges are blurred. The appearance is consistent with myelinated nerve fibres, a normal but rare variant, not usually of any real significance.'

I knew that patients with myelinated nerve fibres around the disc were often misdiagnosed by GPs and opticians as the potentially very serious papilloedema and given an urgent referral to an ophthalmologist. For a few seconds, I felt so pleased with myself I actually thought he would smile and shake my hand and tell me I was the only candidate to have got the correct diagnosis all day.

Papilloedema is an indication of raised pressure within the brain, usually due to a brain tumour or very high blood pressure or hydrocephalus (excess cerebrospinal fluid). The increased pressure leads to swelling of the nerve fibres and loss of the sharp demarcation normally seen. With papilloedema there are associated small flame haemorrhages, caused through microscopic blood vessels bursting and blood within them leaking out and exudates, or whitish areas in the retina. None of these were to be seen in this lady. He stared back blankly, giving no indication of what he was thinking.

'Is there anything you would like to ask her?'

I knew that he was thinking I'd probably mistake it for papilloedema and if it had been that condition I would ask about the symptoms of a brain tumour, such as headache, if it was worse in the morning, visual disturbance, nausea, vomiting.

'Not really, I said, 'This is a normal variant. It is often mistaken for papilloedema.'

'Are you sure?' he asked.

'I'm certain,' I replied, still looking him in the eye.

He turned away, his expression still giving no indication of whether I was right or wrong.

'Well, it's your decision,' he muttered as we walked away, clearly trying to cast some doubt in my mind.

The next patient sat on the edge of the bed. I introduced myself, shaking his hand. He was in pyjamas, about sixty, obese and bald.

'Please examine his chest.'

I took his right hand. There was some nicotine staining on his right fingers. An early clue.

A hyperinflated 'barrel' chest was very suggestive of chronic lung disease. Emphysema. I noticed some small scars on the chest wall. He'd had chest drains inserted at some point, probably for pneumothoraces. A few wheezes here and there. He appeared to be a typical COPD patient. As I listened to his chest I prepared to present my findings and provisional diagnosis and try to anticipate any questions they might ask.

I'd been told in a chest clinic when I was an SHO in cardiothoracic medicine at Broadgreen that in this sort of patient, an almost diagnostic test was to ask the patient to perform a forced vital capacity expiration, although few doctors ever actually performed the test. A person with normal lungs, if asked to breathe in as deeply as possible and then out as fast as possible, to try and almost empty all the air from their lungs, can do this very quickly, in about one second. In a patient with airflow obstruction, narrowed small airways, this emptying of the lungs can take a far longer time, up to ten seconds or so. I asked him to do this and looked at my watch. I have never worn one, my sister had sent it to me four years earlier for my medical school finals. As if on cue after seven seconds he began to cough and splutter. Again, the examiners said nothing, still giving nothing away.

There were a few spot diagnoses, including lesions on a teenager's leg, necrobiosis lipoidica, associated with diabetes and a patient with mixed mitral valve disease with heart murmurs. I knew I'd done well in spite of them giving me no clues as to how they felt I'd done. The final part of the exam was the viva, twenty minutes during which I'd be asked questions on any topic they chose.

As I'd gone around the various rooms, I'd carried a sheet which I'd given to the examiners to sign. I'd put it down during the short cases. I sat down for the viva.

'Where's your sheet of paper?' one asked.

'Sorry I've left it outside,' I replied.

He clearly wasn't impressed.

'Well, you'd better go and find it, haven't you?' he said, shaking his head and looking at the other examiner.

'Shit,' I thought as I went in search of it.

It took me a few minutes and I went back into the room.

'This simply isn't good enough,' one of them said. 'You have lost and wasted almost five minutes of your time. Not a very good start is it?' I could imagine a sensitive, anxious and more easily stressed candidate bursting into tears if they'd been in my place at that moment. It almost seemed as if they were being deliberately difficult, testing me to see if I'd crack. Passing a postgraduate medical degree is effectively a license to become a consultant in that specialty. They didn't want to allow someone to achieve that if they weren't good enough. The viva went better than I could ever have hoped for. I answered every question correctly and knew my responses were all insightful. When the bell rang, they looked at each other again and one nodded slightly.

'We'll give you a few more minutes, the time you lost at the start,' one said.

After another five minutes, they glanced at each other, and as I stood up to leave, both leaned forward and warmly shook my hand. It was clear I'd passed.

I'd heard about this before. In the final exams at the end of medical school the examiners in general were friendly and you had the feeling they really wanted you to pass. You'd been a student for five years. It had cost the country a lot of money to get you through all that training. They were on your side. This was the opposite, it felt as if they were out to fail you, if they possibly could.

A week or so later, my wife rang me about eight-thirty-one morning when I was in the ICU at Arrowe Park after a busy night on call. I'd passed. I went straight into the operating theatres next door to let a couple of the consultants know. They'd helped and supported me over the last year. One of them, about six months earlier, had taken me to one side saying he and a few of his colleagues were very worried that I was studying and working so hard that they felt that I was at risk of having a nervous breakdown. They knew I was studying hard for the MRCP and FFARCS exams at the same time and we had two small children. I was in a busy job with a lot of nights on call. He advised me that I should take a year off from all studying and give myself a break.

I'd just smiled on hearing this and told him that simply wasn't going to happen. Now it was his turn to smile as he congratulated me and said it was just as well I'd not taken his advice. Next was the FFARCS, the anaesthetic postgraduate exam. MRCP or not, I had to pass that if I wanted to be a consultant anaesthetist. It would have all been for nothing if I couldn't pass that too.

Again, this consisted of written papers first. If you passed them, you went to London for the final part. This consisted of a clinical section where you saw a patient and were then grilled by two examiners. A thirty-minute viva was the final part of the exam. I'd failed it the first time, in January 1987. I was back in July for another go. I'd again passed the written part and it was time for the clinical part. At that time I'd moved from Arrowe Park to Alder Hey Children's Hospital for a six-month post and was half-way through that job in July.

The two examiners introduced me to a sixty-year-old lady. I was asked to take a history and examine her. I had thirty minutes. She had several illnesses, but the main problems were hypertension and valvular heart disease and hypertension. As I spoke to her and examined her I was trying to anticipate the questions that were coming. The examiners were back. One was the professor in Edinburgh.

I presented my history briefly, and my examination findings. One asked about her heart murmurs. I said she had aortic incompetence, the valve was leaking and would soon need to be replaced.

'Would you like to demonstrate some signs of aortic incompetence?'

My six months of cardiology in Broadgreen and all the studying for the MRCP was now put to good use. For the first time ever in an exam I was actually enjoying myself. These examiners were anaesthetists, not physicians and were not even aware of some of the signs I was showing them. I could see they were trying not to laugh. The patient's smile reassured me.

They then asked me about some of the drugs she was on and again I'd anticipated this and had the answers ready. I was asked how I would anaesthetise her for a hip replacement and then the professor moved on to tell me a little story. When he'd been a senior house officer in anaesthetics, he'd been asked to see a merchant seaman who'd gone to the A&E department and had been diagnosed with an acute abdomen, or peritonitis. He needed surgery. Again, through having done the MRCP, I anticipated what was coming. For that exam I'd learnt a list of medical causes of abdominal pain, some of them very rare, like lead poisoning and acute intermittent porphyria. I was wondering if this patient might have had syphilis; one symptom of this is acute severe abdominal pain which can mimic a surgical acute abdomen.

At that point it was only a guess but as he went on I was going over in my head the medical conditions causing abdominal pain similar to the pain caused by a surgical problem requiring an operation. When he finished he asked if I had any thoughts on how I'd anaesthetise the man. I said I was concerned this might not actually be a surgical problem and told him I was wondering if it could be a form of syphilis, Tabes Dorsalis. He glanced at the other examiner. I'd guessed correctly. He had too, as a junior doctor.

The next question was the one I thought would be coming.

'Can you tell me any other medical causes of acute abdominal pain?'

I reeled off about eight other causes, which I'd been rehearsing for the previous few minutes. They then asked about the drugs she was on – several were cardiac and antihypertensives. I knew all the answers again through my preparation for the MRCP and my cardiology job. It couldn't possibly have gone better and again, as in my

MRCP, they both stood up and shook my hand at the end. The final part was the viva which also went well.

At about six pm in the foyer of the Royal College of Surgeons in Lincoln's Inn Fields about forty of us anxiously waited for the results. It was a tradition then that a lady would walk about half-way down the staircase, face the anxious candidates below and read out a list of numbers. If your number was called, you'd passed. I'd been there six months earlier when I'd failed. This time my number was called and I walked through to a large room with three others who'd also passed. The other thirty-four candidates that day had failed. We shared a drink with the examiners as each of them congratulated us. Another hurdle overcome.

Next morning it was back to reality and Alder Hey. Of all the hospitals I have worked in I think that was the busiest. I'd heard from other anaesthetists in Liverpool that it would probably be impossible to get better training in paediatric anaesthesia anywhere else in the world. At the interview for my Liverpool registrar rotation post I had asked that if I was fortunate enough to be successful, could I possibly have the post that started there first. I wanted to get the six months at Alder Hey under my belt as quickly as possible so that once I passed the FFARCS final exam I could apply for a senior registrar job and move further towards my eventual aim of being a consultant. I knew I needed paediatric experience before I had a realistic chance of getting a senior registrar post.

The 'Liverpool Technique' of anaesthesia was known to anaesthetists throughout the world.

In the 1940s two Liverpool anaesthetists, John Halton, known as Jack, and Thomas Cecil Gray, known as Cecil Gray and who would later become the Professor in Liverpool, became involved in pioneering work. Coincidentally, Halton would later work as the senior anaesthetist at Noble's Hospital, from 1948 until 1963, although he still worked part-time in Liverpool too, in dental anaesthesia.

General anaesthesia up until that time required that the patient breathe high concentrations of ether or other inhalation agents in order to achieve relaxation of the muscles of the abdominal wall. This relaxation was needed for abdominal surgery. In 1942 anaesthetist Harold Griffith in Montreal was the first to use a muscle relaxant drug, Intocostrin, during anaesthesia, in very small doses so that the muscles involved with breathing were still able to contract. 'To take the edge off muscle tone', as he put it. This was to revolutionise the practice of anaesthesia. Using a muscle relaxant to paralyse these muscles meant that patients could be kept anaesthetised using less inhalation agent, with fewer side effects from the inhalation agent, in particular respiratory and cardiac depression. Patients would wake from anaesthesia much quicker.

In 1943, as an RAF Officer at Burtonwood, Halton mixed with American airmen at the bomber base. He persuaded one of them to fly over some Intocostrin, a derivative of Curare (a paralysing agent once used by South American Indians as arrow poison used to kill animals), and he used this in his thoracic patients. Working with Gray, they reported their experiences with Tubocurarine, a purified derivative of Intocostrin, in 1946. On March 1st that year Cecil Gray delivered a lecture entitled 'A Milestone in Anaesthesia' at the Royal Society of Medicine in London. Much of anaesthesia today is based on their work. Whereas Griffith's patients breathed during surgery, as the Liverpool technique developed, larger doses of Curare were given so that complete abdominal relaxation was achieved. The patients had to be intubated and ventilated as their breathing muscles were also paralysed. The technique was based on the triad of unconsciousness, analgesia and muscle relaxation.

Dr Gordon Jackson Rees, known to his friends as Jack Rees, was a paediatric anaesthetist at Alder Hey and he too developed the Liverpool Technique in paediatric anaesthesia. In 1937, a Newcastle paediatric anaesthetist, Philip Ayre, invented a breathing circuit for use in children. It became known as the Ayre's T-piece. Jackson Rees later added an open-ended bag to the circuit and this became known as the Jackson Rees modification of the Ayre's T-piece circuit. If the child was breathing spontaneously, the bag would inflate and deflate. If a muscle relaxant drug had been given, the open end of the bag was partly occluded with the little finger, pinching it to stop the anaesthetic gas escaping so that the lungs could be ventilated by hand. There were no valves at all in the breathing circuit as these could potentially become faulty and dangerous. The very low resistance to breathing was essential for very small children.

The circuit has been used around the world ever since. I must have used it thousands of times and, like many others, I always considered it to be a stroke of genius from the two anaesthetists. At Alder Hey I never used a ventilator for a child who'd had a paralysing drug during an anaesthetic. None of the anaesthetists did. These patients were all ventilated by hand throughout the operation, often for many hours. Coincidentally, as part of my senior registrar rotation a year later in Newcastle, I would work in the General Hospital and in the Royal Victoria Infirmary, or RVI, where Ayre had been an anaesthetist.

Anaesthetists from around the world would go to Alder Hey to learn the Liverpool Technique. In 1987 I was following in their footsteps and I felt honoured to be there. I was fortunate to work there with such great paediatric anaesthetists as Gordon Bush and Tony Nightingale as they neared retirement, never forgetting their words of wisdom throughout my own career.

I often think about some of the children I helped to look after during that busy six months. The beautiful six-month-old baby girl who'd been shaken by her father, who was allowed in to see her briefly one evening in tears as I was examining her in the ICU one night. He was handcuffed to a police officer. She had a severe traumatic brain injury and was critically ill and on a ventilator. I still think of her now and then even today and wonder whether she survived and if so, what her life is like now, thirty-three years on.

I heard the whole family were out looking around Liverpool for the uncle of a seven-year-old girl, who was suspected of raping her. The police were desperately trying to find him before they did. She was so brave when I spoke to her on the ward before her operation. I anaesthetised her for surgery to repair her damaged body.

A toddler, aged two, had pulled over a chip pan and the boiling hot oil had burnt his face and neck. For a while he was critically ill on a ventilator for several weeks and I saw him each day as he slowly battled back to health. Thankfully he slowly improved and the prognosis for him was looking good as I ended my six months there.

An eight-year-old girl in ICU with meningococcal septicaemia and meningitis wouldn't let anyone but me take her blood and change her IV cannulas. The nurses would come looking for me and if I was busy in the theatre they would wait until I was free to go to the unit. She had a hemiparesis, a weakness of one side of her body caused by damage to her brain. I still wonder how life turned out for that little girl too and I think of her now and then. My feeling is that she made a good, if not complete, recovery.

A few days later I was in the ICU there when Euan, my friend from medical school and at that time also training in anaesthesia with me, tapped me on the shoulder.

'Your job has just come up in the BMJ'.

The British Medical Journal was where all medical posts were advertised and he'd spotted an ad for three senior registrar rotation posts in Newcastle. I'd told him a few weeks earlier that I'd like to go there so Kerry could be near my parents and sister and it would be nice for them to see our children for the next three years or so.

One of the consultants at Alder Hey told me I definitely wouldn't get a senior registrar post as I was too inexperienced, having only completed just under three years of training in the specialty. She felt it would be a waste of time applying.

At the interview I was asked if I could let the panel know why they should give me one of the jobs when there were other candidates there who had another three or four years training under their belts. I'd anticipated that question coming up and I knew my answer would determine whether or not I'd be offered a post.

I explained that during my year of cardiothoracic medicine, I'd done a lot of work as a locum anaesthetist at Arrowe Park. I hadn't actually stopped giving anaesthetics during that year of medicine. All of the posts I'd held, especially the Alder Hey one, were in very busy hospitals, so I felt that I'd gained a lot of experience. In addition to this, I had also had several letters published in the anaesthetic journals, as well as two academic papers. One paper was published in the British Journal of Hospital Medicine and described how anaesthetists can check that a pacemaker is working prior to giving them an anaesthetic. The other was entitled 'Tactile Orotracheal Tube Placement Test'. This was a new confirmatory test to ensure that the tracheal tube was correctly positioned in the airway, rather than the oesophagus. It had the advantage of being quick, reliable and did not require any anaesthetic equipment - just an index finger.

Finally, studying and passing the MRCP had given me the knowledge I'd have not otherwise gained to enable me to better manage and treat patients in ICU and assess patients preoperatively. I was offered one of the three posts and was due to start at the General in Newcastle on Monday December 1st, 1987.

CHAPTER 8

Newcastle

I was born in my maternal grandmother's house in Stanley, a mining village eight miles from Durham City – I was the middle child of three with an older sister and a younger brother. My grandma died when I was three and my grandad when I was eight, but I have hazy memories of the lovely blue stained glass surrounding the front door and hiding inside a grandfather clock which stood in the hall. There were several coal mines in and around the village, and my grandfathers, my dad and all five uncles had worked in them.

In 1909 there was an explosion in one, the West Stanley Colliery or Burns Pit, as it was more commonly known. When I was around twelve, I recall my paternal grandmother explaining how she was eight at the time and remembered hearing the loud bang as did everyone in the village. They instinctively knew what that meant. One hundred and sixty-eight men and boys died.

About twenty-five years ago, I went to Durham library to do a little research into the disaster and looked at the main newspaper of the time, the Durham Advertiser, on microfilm. There was a front-page account of the tragedy. A week or so later, there was an inside description of the funerals with photos showing the Front Street in Stanley packed with mourners and hearses travelling to the cemetery. A week or two later and there was just the occasional short article about the Burns Pit. Today news of a disaster like this would be flashed around the world in minutes and remain as headlines for months afterwards.

My parents had moved to Sacriston a few weeks after my birth, but if anyone ever asked where I was from, I'd always say Stanley. I'm not sure why – perhaps a feeling

If In Doubt

ingrained into my identity by being born there, having all my cousins there and pride in my dad's work in the coal mines.

In Sacriston, we lived in a semi-detached house. It was so cold in winter that we'd scratch images on the ice on the inside of the windows in the sitting room. The worst mornings were when the chimney sweep was coming and the fire wasn't lit, especially in the winter. We'd huddle round a tiny electric fire eating breakfast, shivering.

Despite small hardships like this, I had a blessed upbringing. Next door were Nick, Mam's cousin, and Thelma, who we called Uncle and Auntie, and Susan, a year younger than me. It was as if I had two lots of parents and when I was a teenager, I spent almost as much time in their house as I did in mine and Susan may as well have been my sister.

My mother was also an expert at making tasty meals from ingredients which cost next to nothing. I think that went back to rationing during the war and learning from watching her own mother cooking.

Treacle pudding, my favourite, was simply suet, flour and water steamed for a couple of hours then sliced with golden syrup poured over it. Currant pudding was served with butter and sugar. Bacon and egg pie, cheese and onion pie or my favourite, corned beef pie made with slices of the tinned meat, mashed potato and onions, were often a main meal with chips.

On Sundays, my siblings and I would wait patiently until the beef had roasted for three or four hours before eating 'fat and bread' with salt. If we were lucky, we might get some of the gooey black stuff which my mam insisted was the 'goodness from the meat.' Sliced potatoes were simply just that, in layers with slices of corned beef and onion and water. She'd put a few rashers of bacon on top and when I once asked why she did that she said it was to give it some flavour. For breakfast in the winter, we'd have bacon fried in dripping, the hot fat poured over the bacon. I liked brown sauce with mine, and we'd mop up the fat with bread. My mam would tell us it would keep us warm on our walk to school in the snow.

As a coal miner, my dad worked as much overtime as he could, often seven days a week as a face-worker, the worst job in the mine. He would be hewing coal by hand in narrow wet seams. Like all the miners my dad must have been tough. When I was about seven, I remember going up to the dentist in the village one evening with the rest of my family. It was winter and snowing. He had a general anaesthetic to have his remaining teeth extracted and as we walked back home down the hill in the dark, he had a scarf over his mouth. We walked behind my mam and dad, trying to shelter from the snow. It was around seven o'clock when we got home.

In 1990, during my first year working as a consultant, I was having a drink with him in a pub one afternoon. I told him this story and he said he'd gone to work a few hours later. He'd caught the bus at about 4am and worked his shift at the coal face. His workmates had teased him as his mouth was bleeding when he tried to chew his jam sandwich for his 'bait' and he couldn't talk properly. He never missed work due to being sick. In those days he wouldn't have been paid if he didn't do his shift.

This was my childhood. We'd climb trees and look for conkers, search for birds' nests, fish in the river and play marbles in the school yard – anything so long as we were outside. We'd play football, knock on the front doors of houses at night then run and hide, and we'd steal tyre valve caps to use as whistles.

After my mother died, my sister found a hand-written little booklet in a drawer in her house in which she'd described the ups and downs there had been in her life. I think she knew the end was nearing when she wrote it. I hadn't really appreciated that she hadn't always had a happy life until I read it. I had it made, with some photos, into a booklet and had a printer in Durham run off and bind about thirty copies for our family and friends.

She described her own earliest memory, being told to be quiet in the house, the one where I was born in Stanley. There'd been a lot of people there at the time. She'd realised years later it was at the time of her brother's funeral. He'd been about thirteen years old then and died from meningitis. She described how her 'father' (not 'dad') had never really shown her any affection. He'd worked as a miner, and she described that he spent a lot of time in the local billiard halls.

Her older brother, Harry, had died on D-Day in Normandy when she was eighteen. She described the day the 'dreaded telegram' arrived, and the curtains being drawn for days after that. In 1978 she eventually went to Benouville Cemetery in France with Aunty Thelma and Uncle Nick and found his grave. Nick told me it had been a very emotional moment for her. By the time she was forty her two brothers and her mother and father were all dead.

For all these reasons, securing my three years of senior registrar training in Newcastle, only a few miles from where I grew up, felt like coming home and I was proud to be back, although it felt strange to hear the Geordie accent again after nine years of being away. Four months after starting this post, our third daughter was born there.

One lunchtime I was due to take over an operating list. I'd been on call the night before and had been in theatre until 3am with a young man who had suffered a severe traumatic brain injury in a motorcycle crash. In addition to some bleeding into the brain itself and skull fractures, he also had a subdural haematoma. Blood had collected between the inside of the skull and the surface of the brain. The pressure from this blood clot can be life-threatening. A craniotomy was performed, where part of the skull is removed and the blood clot evacuated. I had kept him anaesthetised at the end of the operation and taken him to the ICU. The outlook appeared to be grim.

After changing I went into the theatre. The consultant anaesthetist, Dr Marshall, was sitting on a stool looking at the monitors.

'Oh, Hi Keith, good to see you,' he said, standing up and folding the newspaper which lay on the anaesthetic machine work surface, tucking it under his left arm and clasping it against his chest before briskly marching into the anaesthetic room next door. I'd been briefly introduced to him a few days earlier in the ICU. He was due to retire soon after 30 years of working at the General Hospital. He was a well-respected neurosurgical anaesthetist and intensivist. He'd written a book too on neuro-anaesthesia which I had read while studying for the final exam a few years earlier in Liverpool. When I sat that exam I had no experience at all of neuro-or cardiothoracic-anaesthesia, but in the final exam you could still be asked about it in the viva and have questions on it in the two written papers.

The sister in charge of ICU had told me he had almost single-handedly set up the ICU there and was very well thought of by her whole team. It was clear she held him in high regard.

By the end of my first year as a senior registrar in Newcastle, I could see why. During ward rounds in the ICU, I learnt a lot from him about the management of brain-injured patients. This training would go on to serve me well as a consultant on the island, particularly during the world famous TT motorcycle races.

I nodded to the ODP, who I'd worked with for the first time the previous day. Surrounded by the team of surgeons, scrub nurses and sterile trolleys covered in operating equipment, there was no visible sign of the patient. I carefully lifted part of the green sterile drapes and peered into the dark space beneath it. A small child lay face down, anaesthetised as the surgeons tried to remove a tumour from the back of the brain. It looked like a boy, with blond hair. I glanced at the anaesthetic chart. A few drugs had been documented at the start of the operation, but it was blank for the preceding couple of hours.

'How long's it been on'? I asked the ODP.

'About three hours,' they replied.

After a couple of minutes I looked in the adjoining anaesthetic room, which was empty. Back in theatre, I looked at the ODP.

'Where's he gone?' I said. I'd assumed the consultant was in there, perhaps getting me some more drugs before coming back to tell me about the surgery; to give me a proper handover.

'He's gone home I think, or more likely to his allotment,' the ODP replied casually.

I was stunned, I had no idea what drugs had been given or when the next ones were due. For delicate surgery like this, one of the essential parts of the anaesthetic for a neurosurgical procedure like this one is to make sure that there is no sudden coughing on the tracheal tube. A muscle relaxant is given so that the patient is paralysed throughout, but if its effects wear off, the stimulus of the tube will cause coughing. All patients having neurosurgery procedures were intubated to ensure there was a secure airway and each anaesthetist had their own preferred way of securing the tracheal tube. Loss of the airway, especially when the patient was prone with the head fixed in position would be a life-threatening situation. The surgery is carried out using an operating microscope. Sudden movement of the patient can be disastrous, even lethal. I had no idea of any blood loss or the pulse and blood pressure during the last two hours or so. I knew nothing at all about the patient. I wasn't even sure if it was a boy or a girl. The ODP told me he was a three-year-old boy.

This was before the days of electronic record keeping. For the first fifteen years or so of my career these observations were documented on the anaesthetic chart by hand. Today, at the end of the procedure, an electronic record is printed and this is then attached to the patient's anaesthetic record, or stored electronically. However, I can think of several patients where for one reason or another I was unable to obtain the printed record. I recall one concerning case where the coroner became involved. He was surprised to learn that I had no electronic record at all after an eight-hour operation. The technology had failed. For this reason, some anaesthetists still write down their observations as we did many years ago. An accurate record of the vital signs during an anaesthetic is crucial in many situations. In the event of a death or a life-threatening complication where the patient comes to harm, for example, the coroner and lawyers will want to know this information. Without it, the anaesthetist will be in a very difficult position if he or she is then suspected of having been negligent in some way during the anaesthetic. I looked seriously at the ODP.

'Keep an eye,' I said. 'I'll be a few seconds'.

The changing room was next to the theatre. Putting on his jacket, Dr Marshall was preparing to leave.

'Is there anything I need to know about this patient?' I asked, not wishing to sound like I was doubting his professionalism.

'Oh, a three-year-old boy having surgery for a brain tumour, been asleep for about three hours and stable throughout. They'll finish in another hour or two I think?' I asked about the muscle relaxant and he said another top-up dose was due in a few minutes.

The ODP looked up as I went back into theatre.

'I can't believe it,' I said. 'Another few seconds and he'd have left the hospital.'

'You should be honoured, really,' the ODP replied, smiling. 'He was talking about you earlier. He'd heard from a few of his colleagues that you seem to know what you're doing and he knows you've just done six months at Alder Hey Hospital. He trusts you. You should be pleased.'

I did wonder what a coroner would make of a situation like this if something went wrong and I'd taken over care of the patient knowing absolutely nothing about him. Fortunately, the operation went well and the little boy woke up a few minutes after it ended.

Throughout my training, Friday nights in Newcastle were always a hive of activity. No matter what the time of year, the city centre, especially the area around the Bigg Market, was always swarming with revellers, some on stag or hen parties, the Geordie girls famous for wearing the skimpiest of dresses and no jacket no matter how cold the weather.

James was twenty-one, a guitarist who played in a band. He was home for a short break and out enjoying catching up with his old school-friends on the Quayside, the up-and-coming area of nightlife in the town or 'toon' as it was better known to the locals. Inside a popular club, around midnight, he'd become involved in a minor altercation with a stranger and the bouncers had to intervene. In the resulting fracas, he was angrily frogmarched towards the exit before being launched over a balcony by one of the bouncers, about twelve feet above the foyer of the building, and onto the darkening street below, left there to be somebody else's problem.

In a panic, his friends charged out after him to discover his contorted body lying motionless in front of them, unconscious, bleeding from his nose and mouth. Hysterically shouting his name, unable to rouse him, they had called an ambulance and he'd been rushed to the General Hospital a couple of miles away. He remained unconscious and a CT scan confirmed he had a serious head injury.

He'd been anaesthetised and placed on a ventilator and his distraught parents arrived in the ICU just as I came onto the ward to begin my two days of on-call that Saturday morning.

For those like myself, the ICU nurses and doctors, the physiotherapists, who would be in and out of the unit, and even the cleaners, the sight of a patient who has clearly been physically assaulted often has no more effect than a sense of intense sadness. Seeing such gruesome images so regularly seems to have the effect of immunising us from the sense of horror and shock that the relatives of the patient must feel.

Although they'd have been gently primed by a doctor and nurse earlier about the effect the sight of their loved one might have on them, surely nothing could really adequately prepare them. Unconscious, with a labyrinth of tubes and lines attached, syringe drivers slowly feeding sedative and other drugs into his bloodstream, loudly beeping monitors blaring, and surrounded by the hustle and bustle of a busy ICU, it is easy to understand how senses can become overwhelmed.

To any outsider, the whole experience must be a terrifying one, yet the reality is that the whole situation can rapidly become worse still. Often, with no way of accurately predicting the likely outcome for the patient, the family are left reeling and pleading for the answers to questions that simply can't be answered. With a potentially serious head injury, there is an immediate dilemma for the doctors and nurses. How do they explain the fact that they can't guarantee how the patient might do in many cases? Surely, with the scans we now have at our disposal, we must know what will happen? Wrong. We know what *could* happen but may not know for sure what *will* happen. That uncertainty can be torturous. Traumatic brain injuries are often caused by road traffic accidents, falls and violent incidents.

Another type of brain injury is hypoxic encephalopathy. This occurs when a lack of oxygen delivered to the brain causes the cells there to die, such as during an out-of-hospital cardiac arrest. Bystander Cardio-Respiratory Resuscitation (CPR), may have been started and continued with the arrival of the emergency services but this may not have been enough to ensure there was an adequate amount of oxygen passing through the lungs into the blood and finally being delivered to the brain cells. The patient would be ventilated in the ICU and sedated, and after a day or two the sedation is stopped so that the neurological status can be confirmed. The concern is always that they may have suffered a catastrophic brain injury through lack of oxygen during the arrest. If the patient does not awaken, the outlook is usually very poor, with death after days or weeks the usual outcome or, worse still in many ways, the condition where they remain unconscious for the rest of their lives but continue to breathe, a persistent vegetative state.

Another common cause for a brain injury, subarachnoid haemorrhage, occurs when an aneurysm, a weakness in the wall of an artery in the brain, suddenly ruptures and blood, under high pressure, spreads around the brain and squashes it. This increased pressure within the brain can cause neurological deficit or brain death. There is often no warning sign and anyone, no matter how physically fit, can suddenly suffer this type of brain bleed. I think most nurses or doctors, when looking after such a patient, think the same as I do: this could be me, or a member of my family lying there instead of the patient, and that thought always stops me in my tracks, seeing the fragility of life in this way.

These patients make up a large percentage of cases who go on to have their organs harvested for donation. The presence of irreversible brain death, after confirmation by a set of tests carried out by two doctors, prompts the search for contraindications for organ donation. James' neurological state was stable by lunchtime, with his pupils still briskly reacting when dazzled by the pen-torch. But then, slowly, a tell-tale worrying sign or two began to appear. Slightly unequal pupils now, not constricting as rapidly as before. Some abnormal posturing, which can be seen when the pressure within the brain rises, arms now extending rather than flexing to a painful stimulus, a pinching of the fingertips. And then there might be the appearance of some ectopic, or extra beats and short runs of a very fast heart rate lasting only seconds, up to one hundred and fifty beats per minute and rising blood pressure.

As the pressure inside the rigid skull increases, known as intracranial pressure, the part of the brain which controls all the vital functions in the brainstem, the respiratory centre controlling breathing and the vasomotor centre controlling the heart becomes compressed, its blood supply reduced. Now it is unable to function correctly. The blood supply to the entire brain is being compromised too because of the high resistance in the blood vessels, again caused by the high pressure. The whole brain begins to die, or infarct, although the heart continues to beat.

His parents were still keeping vigil, his mother slumped forward, exhausted, her head resting on the bed next to his right hand, eyes closed.

A nurse takes me to one side and leans forward to whisper, 'His pupils aren't reacting.' As if hearing its cue, the alarm on the ECG screen now announces another problem, forcing his mother to sit bolt upright and stare ahead, tormented by the shrill ringing of the monitor. The heart rate had shot up to one hundred and seventy beats per minute from a steady sixty, the blood pressure alarm following seconds later, as the figures flash on and off in vivid red, sixty over forty-four, severe hypotension.

There is little doubt now. He is in the process of coning. This is the term given to the condition where part of the brain is forced through a small opening at the skull base, the foramen magnum, by the pressure and swelling, where the brain meets the spinal cord. Irreversible damage occurs to the brainstem containing the vital life-preserving centres. It is happening at that very moment. It's clear now that soon he will be brain dead. It's time for another talk with his parents and they follow me into the visitors' room. In these situations, it is essential that a nurse is present to witness, and later document, what has been said.

They reassure the relatives that in whatever may lie ahead, the comfort and dignity of the patient will always be maintained. Breaking this sort of news has, to me, always been one of the most difficult aspects of my job. It would, of course, not be considered professional for a doctor or nurse to break down and shed tears when they are supposed to be offering support to others in heart-breaking situations like this. How can they do that if they themselves become so upset?

But we are all human. While empathising, that very fine line between maintaining just that exact amount of distancing required to ensure that we don't ourselves break down emotionally, and at the same ensuring that they know we care is very difficult, especially when the patient is a child.

Over the last few years the raised awareness of sepsis has had an impact on the number of deaths due to this cause. Reminders of the early signs are displayed on ambulances and in GP waiting rooms. When a child has meningococcal septicaemia, the onset and deterioration can be so rapid that while involved in the resuscitation it is impossible to resist the feeling that whatever is done, death is almost certain. I have seen it on maybe ten occasions in my career. The illness is so severe and overwhelming that although you press on, going through the motions of putting in IV lines, syringing in boluses of fluid, antibiotics, drugs such as adrenaline to support the circulation, intubating and ventilating, it is impossible to stop the bleak thought creeping into your consciousness. Death is inevitable in many cases.

I had this same feeling when resuscitating a toddler in Liverpool whose mother hadn't noticed when she'd wandered outside one afternoon. She'd found her daughter face down in the garden pond, unconscious and not breathing. Dead. The ambulance had taken about ten minutes to get there and a further twenty to get her into hospital. I intubated her and squeezed oxygen into her tiny lungs, ensuring as best I could that the chest compressions were as effective as possible. We followed the cardiac arrest protocol as her desperate mother stood nearby and watched, tears spilling over in unchecked waves, the comforting arm of a nurse wrapped gently around her shoulders, but we all knew it was futile – even her.

Saying the words, 'We have to stop,' during a resuscitation when the consensus of those involved is that further efforts would be futile is difficult. These feelings are magnified when a child is involved. When we did eventually step back, her mother had seen that we had done all we could for her little girl and thanked us. The agony she must have felt at that moment is unimaginable, but our own sadness was palpable too, and it is often hard to remain composed in such a situation. You can't help but think, 'At least she has seen our struggle with her own eyes.' She knew we'd all tried our best, and in some way that hopefully might have helped her in some small way. We all have a job to do, but when the outcome is not a positive one, the sense of failure can lie heavy on any doctor or nurse.

Now, talking with James' parents is the first step of a journey that will inevitably end in his death. I explain that they already know from his scan that he has a serious brain injury, and that the brain can swell in much the same way a bump appears when we get a 'bang on the head' or sprain an ankle. Being enclosed in an inflexible box, the swelling leads to an increase in pressure and this impedes the blood flow, so the brain cells quickly die. From what we have seen on the CT scan, I think this may be the case, but I need to confirm if this is so by carrying out some tests on him with a colleague. The prognosis is unfortunately very bad and I am sorry. I ask if they have any questions, but, forlornly, they shake their heads, hugging each other and looking at the floor, knowing they would not be offered the words of hope they craved.

I ring a consultant colleague, requesting his help. We carry out tests to establish whether there is any brainstem function, among them: looking for a pupillary response to bright light and a gag reflex or grimace following a painful stimulus, a firm sternal rub using a clenched fist to cause pressure over the breastbone. The most important check is the apnoea test where the tracheal tube, his artificial airway, is disconnected from the ventilator and we watch closely to see if there is any chest movement, indicating breathing. There is none. He is brain dead.

I return to the visitors' room with the same nurse to explain our findings, but there is no reaction to this news; they already know. They both go to speak at once, then stop at the same time, then silence. They look at each other, his father nodding to his wife,

'You tell him.'

'He told us if anything like this ever happened to him we were to make sure his organs were donated. He made sure his name was on the register too. Obviously, we never thought…' Her voice trailed off.

'We need to let the coroner know, but I'll ask him. I'm sure that will be fine,' I say gently. 'I'm sorry,' I said as I got up to leave. I can't think of anything else to say. The nurse stays behind to explain what the process would be from there.

I contact the transplant coordinator. Her job will essentially be to take things from there, arrange for surgeons to come to the hospital to remove his organs, probably the kidneys, heart and liver. She will ensure that any requests from them are answered, measure his chest and heart on his chest X-ray, order blood tests for his blood group and tissue type and arrange transport if this was required for the visiting team. She'll also ask the ICU nurse to let the operating theatre know they would need to prepare for the organ harvest in about six hours.

Before any organ donation can take place, permission must be requested and granted by a coroner. I'm put through to the coroner and begin explaining the situation – the assault and his present condition, and his mother's request. I've already realised there might be a problem.

'I can't allow organs to be taken I'm afraid, this will probably be a manslaughter case, possibly even a murder investigation and we'll need a post-mortem.'

I'd anticipated this.

'He only has a head injury, there's no evidence of any other injury to his body. The transplant surgeons obviously won't be touching the head and neck, could the post-mortem not be carried out later?'

I'm very conscious of the power held by a coroner, so I choose my words carefully.

'Sorry, that isn't acceptable,' he said, with now a vague hint of displeasure, perhaps irritation, in his voice. I need to be very careful.

'Would there be any possibility of trying to have the pathologist who will be carrying out the post-mortem come into theatre so he can watch the organs being taken? He could do an external examination of the body first.'

A pause indicated he was thinking about it.

'No, that won't do either, sorry.'

I don't feel in a position to push it any further and explain this to his parents. His mother sighs and starts to sob softly. The coordinator I've been liaising with, a nurse, arrives in the unit and we are introduced. She is not happy with the coroner's decision but, like me, feels there is little more she can do and goes to briefly chat to his parents, offering her condolences. I say goodbye to them, giving my name and telling them if I can help in any way I would like to. I tell them the coroner's officer will be in touch soon and will need details about their son to pass on to the coroner, who will then prepare for an inquest. Other nurses have heard about what is happening and one by one they come to talk.

'This is awful, isn't it? It's bad enough, but if they can't even get the organs, it's even worse for his parents.'

About an hour later, still in ICU examining another patient, my pager bleeps again; the switchboard operator has the coroner on the phone.

'I was thinking about what you said earlier, and I've been ringing around talking to some other coroners. You are right,' he says.

'Talk to the pathologist and tell him I've given permission to allow organ donation. If he wants to ring me, that will be fine, maybe to discuss whether he feels he should go into theatre or whatever.'

I'm stunned and pause for a few seconds.

'It's too late now. I turned the ventilator off two hours ago after his parents left – he's being prepared for the mortuary.' Organising this procedure takes time, during which the patient must be kept alive on the ventilator - heart beating. Once the heart stops and the organs aren't being perfused with oxygenated blood, they rapidly fail and die making them unsuitable for transplantation.

His turn for a few seconds of silence.

'I'm sorry about that,' he says, then hangs up. I can sense that he recognises a chance has been lost. The nurses are furious, and when I ring the coordinator, she is too.

'We need to do something to stop this happening again,' she declares, and she intends to write to the coroner and ask him to take steps to clarify the situation with other coroners as soon as possible.

One of the saddest incidents relating to organ donation that I was involved with also occurred during this period in Newcastle. The final six months of my SR rotation was in cardiothoracic anaesthesia in the Freeman Hospital. A thirty-five year old, Emma, a lady with two daughters aged fifteen and twelve, had presented with worsening shortness of breath and was found to have a condition known as cardiomyopathy. There are various causes, but in her case it was idiopathic – cause unknown. After diagnosis, the shortness of breath had rapidly worsened over the course of the following year until she was severely breathless at rest. She was dying from heart failure. The only possible option was a heart transplant. Transplants usually took place during the evening and into the night. One evening when I was on call, a possible donor had been found for her. Emma was brought into the anaesthetic room and the preparation for surgery began. Working alongside my consultant, we inserted lines into the neck, an arterial line into the radial artery at the wrist and prepared the drugs we would need for the operation. One of the scrub nurses inserted a urinary catheter. As we were doing this, next door in the operating theatre, the pump technicians, who looked after the cardiac bypass machine, were also busy setting up their own equipment.

While all this was going on, the transplant coordinator was liaising with the team who were carrying out the organ retrieval in a hospital about thirty miles away. Sitting in the coffee room, we chatted whilst we waited for news from the other team. After about twenty minutes, the co-ordinator came in with bad news.

'Sorry,' she said, 'but I've just been informed that the heart is unsuitable.'

The operation was off. Having measured the pressures inside the heart while it was still beating, and watching it closely for a few minutes, they had concluded it would not be acceptable. They couldn't subject the donor to all the risks of this type of major surgery when there was serious doubt about the quality of the new heart. The mood in the room changed and one by one the others drifted off leaving the ODP and me alone in the room.

After about fifteen minutes, the thought suddenly occurred to me that the patient may not yet know that surgery would not be going ahead. I paged the consultant surgeon, who was by now on his way home. Shortly after, he called from home and I asked whether anyone in his team had passed on the news to the patient. After a few seconds he realised that no one had told her and asked if I would explain to her what had happened.

I walked back into the anaesthetic room, having paused outside to compose the right words, but I knew that nothing I could say would make her situation any better. Her chances of survival without this transplant were minimal. This was probably her last chance to live. As I walked into the room, she was sharing a joke with the nurse from the ward and her two daughters.

'I'm really sorry,' I told her, 'but the heart wasn't suitable and we can't go ahead with the operation.' On hearing the news, the young daughters started crying immediately and both hugged their mother tightly. The nurse was close to tears herself.

The ODP and I removed the lines in her wrist and neck and the nurse removed the urinary catheter. When all that was done, she was wheeled out by her eldest daughter – the nurse comforting her other daughter, and back to the ward. I never found out what happened to her, but thought it very unlikely she would live much longer.

Later in my career, during my years as a consultant on the Isle of Man, I'd often need to discuss cases with the coroner. It might be to discuss a patient who had died in ICU and I would ask if he needed further information. A strange sort of black humour ritual went on for years between us each time I rang him. It would go something like this: I'd ask the switchboard to put me through to him. He might be in court, and if so a note would come back from his secretary, telling me she'd pass on my message, then he'd ring back. My bleep would go off and the switchboard operator would say,

'I have the coroner wanting to speak to you, please.'

It was always the same sequence. Silence. I'd press the receiver to my ear listening for breathing, anything. I knew he was there. Then, quietly, in his low-toned voice of authority, slowly, he'd ask,

'Come on now, Keith. Who have you killed now?'

A dilemma. If I laughed, he might say, 'Do you think this is funny?' and tell me off for being rude and disrespectful. If I didn't laugh, he might think I was ignorant for not going along with his bizarre little running joke. I never laughed. I just waited for a few seconds, then started to tell him about my patient.

On another occasion, a twenty-three-year-old man had been in a horrific accident on a farm, sustaining a traumatic brain injury and very severe chest injuries, as well as injuries to his arm, which resulted in it being amputated about two weeks after his admission. He'd been on a ventilator for a month before he died. The large family had taken it in turns to sit by him throughout. They were, understandably, visibly upset when they were informed that the coroner had said he needed a post-mortem.

'He's been through enough,' they said, and I had to agree with them.

I rang him and explained this, asking if a post-mortem examination was really necessary. I knew that, as always, the decision was his alone. To me, there was absolutely no doubt as to the cause of death: multiple organ failure due to multiple trauma including a severe traumatic brain injury and sepsis. He'd had numerous scans and other investigations during his stay in ICU which allowed us to be certain. The coroner told me he felt a post-mortem was essential because of the unusual circumstances surrounding the accident. He was sorry, but this was the reality. I told his family who were upset, but knew I'd at least tried, and they thanked me and left. About two hours later, the coroner rang back. As with the patient mentioned earlier, he'd been speaking on the phone with other coroners in England. He told me he was now satisfied that a post-mortem was not really required. He thanked me for being concerned about the family and prompting him to rethink his decision.

Coroners investigate all deaths that don't have either an obvious or a natural cause. I've always felt they have a very difficult job that carries with it a huge responsibility and I've always had the utmost respect for the work they do. I rang his mother to let her know and she later sent me a heartfelt letter thanking me.

CHAPTER 9

Mistakes

To err is human, to forgive divine.

That may be so, unless you happen to be a doctor and the patient or the patient's relatives haven't heard that particular quote.

Looking back over my career of thirty-eight years, the worst part of it and certainly one of the most upsetting, is that when a mistake has been made, there may be bad feelings afterwards that might last indefinitely. The patient, or their family, may believe that they have been let down so badly that there needs to be some form of compensation for them and also punishment for the doctor.

I have seen many situations when there is no question that a serious error of judgment has occurred. In the vast majority of cases this resulted in no lasting harm to the patient, but in a few, the mistake has led to the patient's death. Whether or not a serious lapse of judgment results in the doctor being called to account depends on a number of factors. These are only my own views, but I have thought about this sort of scenario a lot over the years and I believe that many doctors would agree that they are reasonable and fair ones.

If, prior to the mistake being made, there was a good relationship between patient and doctor, I feel the tendency for the patient to immediately feel that a complaint is justified is diminished. If the doctor, whether he or she was a surgeon, obstetrician or anaesthetist, or whoever appeared to be genuinely concerned, upset even, and had been polite before the incident occurred and apologises after it, they may feel less inclined to complain formally to the hospital complaints department, or even the GMC.

Any of these would upset a doctor, especially the latter one. I feel one of the most important things is an apology by the doctor if he or she feels they have made a mistake. This might not prevent a complaint being made and an investigation and possibly even a visit to a GMC disciplinary hearing, but being open and admitting to the patient a mistake has been made is, to me at least, the right thing to do.

I'm sure one of the things that patients hate more than anything is any hint of a cover-up by the doctor themselves or other doctors who may be perceived to be helping protect the reputation of one of their own. 'Doctors closing ranks' is a term I have heard on a few occasions.

Any doctor who comes across as arrogant, rude, impatient and worst of all, uncaring, is laying him or herself open to a complaint. Another important factor in whether a complaint might be made is whether or not there are close relatives. If a patient has died and had lived alone with no close family, there may be no one to complain.

I was asked to become involved in the care of a seventy-six-year-old man who had developed complications following a relatively minor procedure to remove a rectal polyp. He'd developed severe abdominal pain, vomiting and shoulder pain which suggested a probable leak at the site of surgery. Gas under the diaphragm seen on the chest X-ray confirmed this. Gas, along with some of the contents of the rectum, had passed into the peritoneal cavity. He was taken back to theatre three days after the first operation and was also found to have an area of gangrenous bowel which was excised.

Gas under the diaphragm often leads to transmitted pain which is felt in the shoulders. This is sometimes seen after laparoscopic surgery. During this procedure carbon dioxide is passed into the peritoneal cavity to create a space so that the surgeon is able to operate. At the end of the operation the surgeon tries to remove as much of the gas as possible to minimise the risk of this type of postoperative pain.

If In Doubt

All the clues had been there to indicate that he was seriously ill with peritonitis and septic shock. The surgeon had not recognised this until it was too late, and the patient died in the ICU the day after his second operation. I told his son I was sorry but to me his father had been let down badly. He should have been taken back to theatre much earlier.

'I'm sure they all did their best', he said.

It was clear that he had no intention of complaining. I told the surgeon I felt he'd been very lucky. If a complaint had been made it was very likely that the coroner would have informed the GMC. The patient's son told the coroner's officer that he was satisfied with his father's care. No inquest was held, and the coroner gave permission for the death certificate to be issued. If the family of a patient who died under similar circumstances were not so understanding or sympathetic then the ball would start rolling towards an inquest, possible GMC intervention and all the repercussions that might mean for the surgeon.

In some cases the police can become involved and there are many cases in which a doctor's actions, or lack of action, have led to a manslaughter charge being levelled. Most doctors go into the profession because they want to help others in need and they can empathise with patients and gain satisfaction from being able to do this. I have always felt that whenever I read about a doctor who is in trouble in this way, I ask myself,

'Could that be me?' and invariably the answer is usually a resounding,

'Yes, of course it could.'

Bob Wilkes, one of the consultant anaesthetists in the Royal in Liverpool during my first year of training told me, 'You are only as good as your last anaesthetic,' and I've never forgotten that. Four years later he gave me a reference for a senior registrar post. I got the job and on my last day working in Liverpool I went to see him to thank him for the reference and everything he'd taught me. I asked if he had any advice. He replied, 'Don't change'. I'm fairly certain in saying this he meant that just because I would be a senior registrar and then a consultant, I shouldn't let it go to my head. No matter what or who you are, you can still make a mistake. I personally feel that just about any doctor if given the right set of circumstances is at risk of having some serious complications. We are all human and can all make mistakes.

Jennie Hunter was another excellent anaesthetist I learnt a lot from during my first year. She was one of those rare doctors who was good at everything and highly respected. As well as being an academic researcher and a lecturer in the Department of Anaesthesia, she was involved in the care of ICU patients and would also anaesthetise patients in theatre.

Jennie was funny as well as being an excellent teacher. Over the next twenty-five years or so I'd occasionally see her at anaesthetic meetings. She would become an examiner for the final exam and the first woman to become Editor-in-Chief of the BJA, the British Journal of Anaesthesia. She was also Honorary Secretary of the Anaesthetic Research Society. As with Bob Wilkes, I owe a lot to her.

For all anaesthetists there are certain well-known anaesthetic disasters waiting in the wings and ready to strike. Although perhaps hard to understand by the lay public, a tracheal tube which has been inadvertently placed in the oesophagus instead of the windpipe so that no oxygen enters the lungs, still occurs today and can result in death or severe brain damage.

A case of this happened in my first year of anaesthetic training in Liverpool. A patient was anaesthetised for an appendicectomy. An SHO, like me in his first year of training, had intubated the patient.

He found it difficult to ventilate her and suspected bronchospasm, or constriction of the small airways identical to that which occurs during an asthma attack. This can happen when the patient has a reaction to one of the injected drugs, often a muscle relaxant. These are given to paralyse the abdominal muscles so as to make the operation easier for the surgeon, and they also paralyse the vocal cords so that placing the tracheal tube is easier. Without this, the cords would close to protect the airway and this would make intubation very difficult.

An anaphylactic reaction was suspected. This occurs when chemicals released when the body reacts abnormally to a drug cause airway constriction, like an asthma attack, also a skin rash, increase in heart rate and a drop in the blood pressure and in serious cases this can rapidly lead to the patient's death if not managed swiftly. It usually responds to stopping the drug, steroids, an antihistamine, intravenous fluids and in severe cases, adrenaline.

Help was summoned and the consultant anaesthetist who arrived suspected that the tracheal tube might be in the oesophagus. He'd asked the SHO if there was any possibility of this and was told it was definitely correctly positioned. The consultant then made his fatal mistake – he accepted this answer without checking for himself. By this time, the patient had suffered a cardiac arrest and resuscitation was in progress. Suddenly, green fluid from the stomach, gastric juice, appeared in the breathing circuit and it was instantly clear that the tube was not in the trachea. It was immediately removed and re-inserted correctly into the airway. By then it was too late and the patient had died.

The consultant had been criticised by the coroner at the subsequent inquest for accepting the word of a very inexperienced anaesthetist. He hadn't followed the adage that all anaesthetists know when faced with this sort of situation: *'If in doubt, take it out.'* This is an old dictum for tracheal intubation. An unrecognised oesophageal intubation will inevitably lead to death or a hypoxic brain injury due to lack of oxygen

Litigation, being sued, is a worry that all doctors have. Things don't always go to plan and there are recognised risks. Complications can occur through no fault of anyone, but what happens next depends a lot on the patient as described above.

Being questioned by police during an investigation into a death and the possibility of actually being charged with manslaughter must be a terrifying prospect for any doctor who has never been in trouble before. If found guilty, there might be a custodial sentence. The GMC would become involved and would probably either suspend the doctor's licence to practice for a period or might even strike him or her off the medical register. Erasure from the GMC register would probably signal the end of the doctor's career, although they can in some cases be reinstated.

Anaesthetists are in a specialty which has a relatively high incidence of litigation when compared to other medical specialties. From relatively minor complaints, such as a damaged tooth or crown, to a death under anaesthesia, there is always the spectre of litigation. I have found that almost all of the hundreds of doctors I've worked with, thousands even, are good people who want the best for their patients. They get upset too when things don't go as well as they would have liked and apologise and try to be as honest as possible with their patients. As with any line of work, there are always going to some who seem to lack empathy and compassion. Thankfully, in my experience, they are a minority.

Looking back now, I can recall several incidents when I made a mistake. One was during an operation when I was a registrar. A twenty-five-year-old young lady was having a submandibular gland removed. For various reasons the operating list had over-ran and instead of finishing around five thirty, it was around eight pm when we started this operation, the last one on the list. I'd not had a break all day and was tired and in retrospect I should have said it was late and the patient would have to be cancelled. The operation lasted an hour or so and at the end I extubated her.

A few seconds later, the suction bottle attached to the drain in the wound started to rapidly fill. A suture on an artery had slipped off due to the suction and the escaping arterial blood was being sucked into the drain. The wound needed to be re-explored immediately and I quickly reintubated the patient and the surgeon started to reopen the wound.

In those days, we didn't have pulse oximeters which give a continuous display of oxygen levels in the blood. Their use became routine very shortly after this incident. After a few minutes, the surgeon commented that the blood 'looked a bit blue' and I walked round the table and lifted the surgical drape to look at the fingers. They were blue too. I'd accidentally put the tube in the oesophagus. I asked the surgeon to stop, removed the tube and inserted it into the trachea. No harm had been done but it could have had very serious implications.

Of all of the serious anaesthetic complications I have read about over many years, one in particular stands out. It would be almost impossible to imagine a worse scenario than one which occurred in 2002 and was widely reported in the press at the time. A healthy baby died while having a relatively minor procedure for pyloric stenosis.

Pyloric stenosis in babies occurs when there is an obstruction to the outflow from the stomach caused by a thickening of the muscle layer. This leads to projectile vomiting and it occurs in babies around the age of six weeks to three months and is more common in boys.

Surgery for this is relatively simple: pyloromyotomy. The thickened muscle is carefully divided down to the mucosa, the lining of the pylorus. The commonest complication is causing a small leak in the mucosa, the lining of the junction of stomach and duodenum, the pylorus. This can lead to peritonitis.

I have anaesthetised around fifteen babies for this procedure during my career and in one this complication occurred, about fifteen years ago. The day after surgery, it became clear that the baby had peritonitis and, accompanied by a nurse, I took him to Alder Hey by air ambulance after some IV fluid resuscitation and analgesia had been given. When we arrived in the unit, I handed him over to a nurse who I'd worked with when I'd been a registrar there about eighteen years earlier. She jokingly asked why we had brought a perfectly normal baby in a little plane all the way to Liverpool from the Isle of Man. I told her there was no question in my mind that he had peritonitis and he needed surgery. The reason he now appeared normal was because of the treatment he had received, the IV fluid and analgesia, which were masking the underlying problem.

I rang the ward at Alder Hey the following morning to enquire how he was. The same nurse told me the surgeons hadn't been convinced either, so they'd observed him carefully for about four hours before it became clear that he was in pain from peritonitis and this was causing his breathing to become laboured. He'd then been taken to theatre where the leak was confirmed, repaired and the peritoneal cavity lavaged, or washed out. He made a rapid recovery.

At the end of surgery for pyloric stenosis, known as a pyloromyotomy, the surgeon, before closing the abdomen, often looks for any leak in the mucosa by first flooding the peritoneal cavity with warm fluid. They then ask the anaesthetist to inject air into the stomach through the nasogastric tube while watching for any bubbles which would signify a leak. This would then have to be repaired in order to prevent peritonitis. In the tragic case in 2002 the anaesthetist injected twenty ccs of air into a three-way tap from a syringe while the surgeon looked for the tell-tale bubbles. The stomach had not distended with air so he asked for more air to be injected into the nasogastric tube. At this point, the baby suffered a cardiac arrest and it was realised that air had been accidentally injected into the intravenous line into the blood instead of into the tube in his stomach causing a massive air embolism. The baby died and the anaesthetist was charged with manslaughter.

At trial, his colleagues provided character references. One said he would still be more than happy for the defendant to anaesthetise his own children for any procedure. He had anaesthetised for around forty such procedures and was an experienced consultant anaesthetist. At the end of the trial, he was found not guilty.

In the moments after the baby suffered the cardiac arrest, he would have known what lay ahead. Understandably, there would be angry, unforgiving parents, a hospital and police investigation, a GMC disciplinary hearing, possibly being struck off, a charge of manslaughter and a possible prison sentence and the end of his career. Worse than all of this would, to me, be the feeling of guilt and having to live with this for the rest of his life.

A momentary lapse of concentration had led to the death of a healthy baby and I knew immediately when I read about the case that I could have done what the anaesthetist involved did and I felt sympathy for what he must be going through. He hadn't deliberately set out to cause the death, he'd made a terrible mistake.

When I was in Liverpool an anaesthetist made a mistake during an elective operation and a woman of about thirty died. Her husband sued the hospital and the case dragged on for several years. The anaesthetist later committed suicide, leaving a note explaining the guilt he felt and apologising. I recall reading an article in the local newspaper. The husband of the woman who died said he'd never wanted that to happen and tragically now he'd lost his wife and the anaesthetist's wife had lost her husband.

One of the worst possible situations for an anaesthetist is one in which it proves impossible to be able to ventilate or intubate a patient. If an unconscious patient is breathing but has an obstructed airway, they require an airway opening manoeuvre, a chin lift or jaw thrust. This may be all that is required apart from giving oxygen via a face mask. An adjunct, such as an oropharyngeal airway, can be inserted to maintain the patency of the airway. If the patient is not breathing adequately once the airway has been opened, or is not breathing at all, they require ventilation with oxygen with a bag-valve mask device. If a patient can't be ventilated in this way, they require tracheal intubation. If this proves impossible too, the last resort is a cricothyroidotomy.

This procedure allows oxygen to enter the trachea via the front of the neck, via a plastic cannula inserted over a needle or, better still, via a small tube placed through a surgical incision. This situation, very rare, is known as a 'can't ventilate, can't intubate' scenario. In my whole career I have had to do this only three times.

About ten years ago, I was to anaesthetise for an ENT list. There were quite a few patients on the list and for some reason I was running a bit late at the start, so I asked that the first one be sent for and I would just see her in the anaesthetic room instead of on the ward to save a little time. Most patients on this list were usually fit and low risk for any anaesthetic complications. She was about forty years old, generally well and was due to have a general anaesthetic for tonsillectomy.

I asked about previous anaesthetics and she said there had been some problems when she'd had surgery in Scotland a few years back for a sterilisation, but was very vague about this. She'd been told they had struggled to insert a tube into her airway. As a teenager her mother had told her that she had a congenital abnormality of her neck, with two or three of her cervical vertebrae fused, rather than separate bones. This can lead to restricted mobility of the cervical spine and make tracheal intubation difficult.

I briefly examined her upper airway and neck movements. There was some restriction in neck mobility but I wasn't particularly concerned about this. I told her that I probably wouldn't need to intubate her anyway as I had planned to use a flexible laryngeal mask instead. I didn't preoxygenate her. This is where the patient breathes 100% oxygen for a minute or two prior to being anaesthetised. The lungs become filled with oxygen so that in the event of there being an airway problem immediately after consciousness is lost – where it is difficult or impossible to ventilate with a face mask, there will be a longer period before the patient becomes hypoxic. The extra oxygen reservoir in the lungs resulting from preoxygenation buys time for the anaesthetist. This can be life-saving in some very rare situations.

I anaesthetised her and quickly realised I was in trouble. Her airway became immediately completely obstructed. I performed airway opening manoeuvres, a chin lift and jaw thrust. In almost all patients these are successful in opening an obstructed airway and allow oxygen to be given. Both were totally ineffective.

I tried to bag her with the anaesthetic breathing system, but without success. Insertion of an oropharyngeal airway then a nasal airway was also unsuccessful. It was still impossible to open her airway and ventilate and by now she was cyanosed, the alarm on the pulse oximeter beeping. She would have a hypoxic cardiac arrest soon, her heart would stop because it was so lacking in oxygen.

Next, I tried a laryngeal mask and this too proved useless, so I carried out a laryngoscopy, looking with a laryngoscope to see if I thought there was a chance of intubating her. I was unable to see any of the vocal cords and knew I'd never be able to insert a tube by using any other type of scope in the next few seconds. There simply wasn't time. She'd become too hypoxic.

This was now the scenario feared by all anaesthetists: 'Can't intubate, can't ventilate.'

In retrospect I should have given a small dose of an induction agent then checked to see if I could ventilate with a face mask. That would have proved impossible but she would then have woken up a lot quicker so the risk of losing the airway for a longer period would have been reduced. I realised it would be six or seven minutes until she recovered from the dose I had given her. I told the ODP that this was now a life-threatening situation and I needed to perform a needle cricothyroidotomy as soon as possible so that I could oxygenate her. This involves passing a cannula over a needle inserted through the skin over front of the neck, and through the cricothyroid membrane and into the airway. Oxygen can then pass through the cannula and into the lungs. Within seconds, while I was inserting the needle and aspirating air to ensure that it was in the airway, he had connected a Sanders injector to the back of the anaesthetic machine. This is used during rigid bronchoscopy, a procedure used to diagnose and treat lung conditions. The anaesthetist can then 'jet' oxygen at very high pressure in short bursts (jets), via the bronchoscope to keep the patient oxygenated while they are being kept anaesthetised by intravenous drugs.

I removed the needle, leaving the cannula in the upper airway and connected the injector. I was extremely relieved to see her cyanosis disappear almost immediately after a few jets of oxygen.

As the effects of the IV anaesthetic induction agent wore off, she started to regain her airway as she started to breathe again. Once I was sure she could maintain her own airway I removed the cannula from the front of her neck.

Later, when she was fully awake in the recovery room, I went to speak to her, explaining that she hadn't had her surgery. There'd been a very serious problem. I apologised to her for not being able to anaesthetise her so she could have her operation. During my whole career she was one of only three patients who'd been given a general anaesthetic and woke up without having had their surgery.

'I knew you wouldn't be able to do it, don't worry,' she said, and didn't appear in the least bit concerned. I explained that she needed to inform any anaesthetist in the future that I'd been unable to ventilate and intubate her and I documented what had happened in the notes. If she required a general anaesthetic again, the safest technique would probably be an 'awake intubation.' This involves inserting the tube using a fibreoptic laryngoscope with the patient awake and maintaining their own airway. It is used when there is a known or suspected difficult airway.

When I later went through the correspondence in the case notes, I came across a letter from an anaesthetist in Scotland who, coincidentally, I had briefly trained with in Liverpool. In it they explained identical problems to the ones I had encountered.

After tracking the anaesthetist down, I rang her. When I gave her the patient's details, she recognised the name immediately and said,

'Shit, we almost killed her!'

I'd almost killed her too. I'd made the very serious mistake of not really going into the detail I should have when she told me there had been issues with her airway during a previous operation. I should have looked through the correspondence. I should have pre-oxygenated her and assessed her airway and cervical spine mobility in more detail. I should have been better prepared for a very difficult airway. During my career there were several occasions where I had to deal with life-threatening airway obstruction. Some occurred as a result of serious facial trauma in an unconscious head injury patient. Others involved laryngeal tumours or a foreign body occluding the upper airway. This incident, however, was by far the most challenging I ever encountered. Fortunately, she'd not come to any harm, but it had been close. She had been lucky and so had I.

I was woken up one morning at about 5am when I was in Newcastle and was told they needed me urgently in A&E at the General Hospital. In a freak accident, a milkman had slipped on ice and landed on a bottle he'd been carrying which broke, the shattered glass slicing into the femoral artery in his groin. He was very pale, shocked, almost white, and had clearly lost a lot of blood. The paramedics had reported a lot of blood at the scene. Several attempts had been made in A&E to gain IV access, including several unsuccessful attempts to cannulate veins in the right side of his neck before the jugular vein on the left side was cannulated and fluid resuscitation was started. Blood was urgently cross-matched, I anaesthetised him, and they began to explore the lacerated artery and repair it with a graft.

As the operation proceeded, I became very concerned. I was as sure as I could be that I'd given enough blood to restore his circulating volume but his blood pressure remained low and his pulse high at around one hundred and twenty per minute. An infusion of Noradrenaline was started which had little effect on the blood pressure. I told the surgeon that something was very wrong but I couldn't work out what was going on. He remained fairly stable for the next four hours until the operation ended and the surgical drapes were removed. As we prepared to take him to the ICU the patient's chest was again revealed. The reason for the hypotension and tachycardia became immediately apparent to me. The right side was barely moving and I listened with a stethoscope. No air entry and a hyper-resonant percussion note: he had a tension pneumothorax.

As I'd been ventilating him after intubation, a tiny amount of the gas had passed into the pleural space with each breath through a tiny hole caused by the desperate attempts earlier to insert a line into his neck when he'd arrived in A&E shocked and peripherally shut down with no other veins visible. The gradual increase in size had then caused the underlying right lung to collapse, effectively having been squashed by the pressure in the air cavity around it, the pneumothorax. This pressure also led to a reduction in the amount of blood returning to the heart via the inferior and superior vena cava veins, sensed by the body as hypovolemia, low blood volume and the heart had reacted with an increase in rate to try to increase the amount being pumped around the body. The clue had been there all along, the small puncture wounds in his neck, but I'd forgotten about them.

With this condition it would be expected that there would also be a very high inflation pressure needed so that the ventilator could force in gas in spite of the high pressure within the chest. In retrospect, it was higher than normal but not dramatically so. Also, one might expect that a high concentration of oxygen might be needed to counteract the effects of the collapsed lung, but this didn't seem to have happened here either.

I quickly inserted a chest drain – there was no need for a chest X-ray to confirm it – to allow the trapped gas to escape and within seconds the right side of his chest started to move normally as the collapsed lung reinflated, the heart rate slowed and blood pressure rapidly increased. Fortunately, my delay in making the diagnosis had not caused him any harm and he made an uneventful recovery.

Mistakes do sometimes happen but in anaesthesia they can have disastrous consequences both for the patient and the anaesthetist, as well as the patient's loved ones. And the loved ones of the anaesthetist.

CHAPTER 10

Clefts

I was watching an episode of Blue Peter about thirty years ago with my daughters and a feature about children having cosmetic surgery for cleft lip and palate surgery came on, I think in Africa.

The team of surgeons, anaesthetists and nurses were moving from place to place by plane, carrying out operations in an operating theatre on a plane. As the filming went on, they were to film one of the last children being taken to the makeshift hospital for his own surgery for a cleft lip repair. The plane would fly them on to their next destination after the mission ended.

The boy, about seven years old, hadn't arrived for his surgery and the film crew went to his home, a wooden hut, to see why he hadn't been taken in by his mother to have the operation. She spoke no English and explained through an interpreter that he had wandered off and she'd been unable to find him. The team were due to fly off to their next destination within hours and there was debate about whether there was time to actually carry out the operation even if they could find him in time.

As I watched this, I felt the suspense building. It was a fantastic feature and I have never forgotten it. The Blue Peter crew and some of the charity team went off to search for him, in a jeep. He was found on his own, idly kicking a tin can around and they essentially snatched him off the street, ignoring his protests and took him for surgery. The programme ended with him waking up from the anaesthetic having had his surgery and being reunited with his mother. I felt very moved by it and still remember telling colleagues at work in the operating theatre the following day.

If In Doubt

It was an incredible story to me as a doctor; what could be more rewarding than this, essentially being part of the team who has given a child a new and beautiful face? Correction of a cleft lip has always seemed to me to be the ultimate corrective plastic surgery procedure. It simply can't be hidden. Everyone sees it immediately. I felt quite moved by it and have never forgotten it.

I'd been involved in some cleft lip and palate surgery while I was at Alder Hey in Liverpool during my training – it was the biggest paediatric hospital in Europe and a regional centre for carrying out this procedure. As a registrar, we would assist the consultant anaesthetists for this type of anaesthetic. Throughout my career I'd been anaesthetising for tonsillectomy, adenoidectomy, dental extractions and some ENT operations in children. Some of this was similar to anaesthesia required for cleft surgery.

For the first fifteen years or so of my consultant work in the Isle of Man I did most of the chair dental anaesthetics. These were short procedures requiring a general anaesthetic, mainly children for dental extractions. At that time, the first ten years or so of my consultant post, there were three main centres where these procedures were carried out; the hospital itself, a secondary school close to the hospital and a dental practice, also close by. I'd take an ODP to assist me.

I'd go to the school on Monday and Wednesday mornings and later, for about eight years, I'd give all the anaesthetics in the dental practice. One morning, we did twenty-one general anaesthetics there, although on average there would be ten to fifteen or so, a few adults, but mainly children. None of the patients for this type of procedure were intubated or had laryngeal masks. They were anaesthetised with a facemask which was removed so the dentist could work in the mouth, or in some longer cases, a nasal mask would be used. It was tricky because I needed to ensure the airway was kept open with a jaw thrust while keeping them anaesthetised with the nasal mask in place and also used a metal mouth gag to keep the mouth open.

Although we never encountered any serious issues, general concerns arose about the safety of this sort of work and it became a requirement, from around 2002, that all such general anaesthetics must be given in hospitals. This type of work would prove to be useful if I ever decided to anaesthetise for cleft palate surgery. Around 2008, I started to look into how I might be able to become involved in some voluntary work myself. I'd been thinking about this on and off since that TV programme.

On the Smile Train website, a charity involved with cleft repair, there was a small article about a US charity, CCK (Community Cares for Kids). Each year three or four consultant plastic surgeons who'd been at medical school together, gave up a week of their time to carry out plastic surgery in Ecuador for a week. At that time, it had been going for about ten years. They took a team of nurses with them for the missions, from Philadelphia and Florida. Through charity events they raised money to pay for the trip, flights and hotel accommodation, and all the equipment and drugs they'd need. Frank Collini, a plastic surgeon in Shavertown, Pennsylvania, had started the charity and I emailed him, explaining I was interested in joining them if this might be possible. It was the start of three missions with his team, the first in 2009.

It didn't get off to a great start. I'd never travelled in Business Class, so I decided as it was a long trip, I'd treat myself. I flew to Guayaquil, with a population of two million, via Madrid and arrived there at four o'clock in the morning. That mission was to take place in a hospital in a naval base in Manta, a coastal resort about one hundred and fifty miles from Guayaquil and I'd been told a naval employee would meet me at the airport and drive me there.

I waited for my bag. Along with my clothes I'd brought some medical equipment; laryngoscopes, tracheal tubes, my stethoscope, breathing circuits and bag-valve-masks and I'd stupidly put eight hundred US dollars in it. As the baggage came off and went round the carousel, I soon realised mine had gone astray. I tried to explain what had happened, but no one spoke English, so after half an hour or so I gave up and made my way out of the arrivals area. A sailor, all in white, met me and gestured, wondering where my bag was. He didn't speak any English as I tried to explain it hadn't arrived with me as I climbed into the back of the car for the one-hundred-and-sixty-mile drive to Manta, a resort on the coast. It was 8.30am when we arrived at the hotel, and I was told my room wouldn't be ready until around 2pm. There was only one solution. I only had ten dollars, but with my card, I managed to get some cash from a machine and I bought a few beers and sat by the pool for an hour before buying shorts, t-shirt and flip flops at a kiosk on the beach. I had the next day, Saturday, to relax before we started work on Sunday. Manta was a seaside resort and the hotel was right next to the beach. The rest of the team arrived late on Saturday evening and I met them briefly at breakfast on Sunday.

Later that morning was triage where the patients were seen by the three surgeons and if suitable for surgery, were next seen by us and listed for their operations. With a nurse to help us we'd try to get a history and examine their heart and chest.

They were nearly all children, but one or two adults had turned up for triage and were listed for these procedures if there was time to do them, some under local anaesthetic. It was decided it might be appropriate to carry out cleft palate surgery on a man of twenty; the rest of the cleft lips and palates were all children. If Frank's team managed to carry out a specific number of cleft procedures they would receive some funding from the Smile Train charity, but some other operations were done as well. One of the team was an orthopaedic surgeon with an interest in congenital bone disorders of the foot, mainly club foot. Some children had cerebral palsy and had tight hamstring muscles making it difficult for them to walk. Tendon release could help them.

At the end of that day the theatre lists for the week were typed up and displayed on a board and the patients' parents, who had been waiting patiently all day, crowded around the theatre lists to see when their child was to have their operation. We were ready to go the following morning. There were three surgeons and four anaesthetists, so there was always one spare in case any help was needed unexpectedly. My initial impression of one of the team, all from the US, was that they were very friendly, though I recall one anaesthetist came across as slightly arrogant – the sort who'd proudly carry a briefcase and wear a raincoat, I thought.

On the second morning I was helping this anaesthetist, Dave, who was working with Frank that day, at the start of his anaesthetic. We'd have two anaesthetists for the cannulation and intubation and, once the airway was secured, the second one would go off to his own theatre to start his case. He'd made a few unwelcome comments about the way I was squeezing a child's hand to get the veins to fill, how I'd inserted an IV cannula and how I'd handed the tracheal tube to him a few times during the first day, and he persisted in making such comments as the morning went on.

He'd even questioned how I squeezed the bag on the breathing circuit when I was ventilating a patient.

Growing irritated, I took him to one side and told him I'd not travelled all that way to have my capabilities as an anaesthetist questioned by him, and he apologised immediately, looking a bit sheepish as he went back to his patient. Two of the theatre nurses came to me later on to say they were pleased that someone had put him in his place as he'd upset a few others too.

Later that day, I wandered into the recovery ward while my next patient was being prepared for theatre.

The man who'd been listed for the cleft palate repair had just had his operation and was sitting up on a bed holding a kidney dish containing blood at chest level. As I watched, he'd lean forward every few minutes and spew out clots of blood into the dish. I asked how long he'd been there and a nurse said it was about an hour. They'd informed the surgeon, but he'd said they needed to be patient and he felt the bleeding would stop soon.

I asked him to open his mouth wide by demonstrating what I meant as he spoke no English. When he did so, I saw that his tongue was grossly swollen and was being pushed up towards the roof of his mouth due to bleeding underneath it. It was clear to me that soon he'd be at risk of complete upper airway obstruction and I asked a nurse to find Frank and tell him he needed to see the patient urgently. It would already be very difficult, if not impossible, to re-intubate him if that happened.

He arrived a minute or so later and I told him the patient needed to go back to theatre urgently before he developed signs of airway obstruction and intubation might then not be possible. I told him I felt he needed to take over and carry out the operation himself. I said this was a potentially very serious, life-threatening situation. The surgeon who did the operation should have realised earlier what was happening.

When he was taken back into the theatre, I could tell that Dave was very worried about the intubation as I prepared the drugs and equipment for him. He asked what I thought he should do and we discussed the safest way forward. The concern was that if he'd been given a paralysing drug, ventilating him with a face mask might be difficult as might intubating him because of his tongue obstructing the view of the cords. Instead, we 'gassed him down,' using an inhalational anaesthetic rather than an intravenous one.

Fortunately, intubation was relatively straightforward and once he was happy, I went back to my own theatre to start my next case. About an hour later Dave came into my theatre and told me the operation had finished.

'What do you think I should do now?' he asked, looking a little embarrassed.

'What do you mean?' I replied. I hadn't understood what he was getting at.

He explained that he was concerned about taking the tube out in case there was a problem with his airway again. He felt there may be swelling of tissue in his upper airway and of the vocal cords which might cause obstruction once the tube was removed. He also knew we couldn't leave the tube and ventilate him overnight because there was no High Dependency Unit or ICU.

I reassured him that I was fairly certain he'd be okay and he asked that I be there when the patient's tracheal tube was taken out. I suggested he have a look with the laryngoscope to see if he could get a good view of the cords and assess the swelling of the tongue. If it looked okay I would sit him up and extubate him when he was almost awake so he could maintain his own airway when the tube came out. I'd suggested earlier that he gave IV Dexamethasone, a steroid, which can reduce swelling of the lining of his upper airway.

Initially after the tube came out the patient appeared to be breathing normally, but after a minute or so he began to struggle and he developed noisy breathing, worse on inspiration, making a crowing sound. He became agitated, moving his head from side to side rapidly and it was clear to me that he had laryngospasm. This occurs when the vocal cords close to protect the upper airway from contamination from blood or vomit in a patient who is semi-conscious. Dave started to panic and started to draw up drugs for reintubation, but I reassured him that it would settle if we waited.

I screwed down the expiratory valve on the breathing circuit filled with 100% oxygen so that if the cords were even slightly open the high pressure would force oxygen into his lungs. It can become a vicious circle; the patient feels he can't breathe because of the cords closing, becomes anxious and the anxiety leads to the laryngospasm becoming even worse until the cords close completely, and the patient then can't breathe in at all. Reassurance verbally is sometimes enough, but a small dose of IV sedation is sometimes needed to break the spasm.

After a minute or two he settled down and the noisy breathing became less and soon disappeared completely. Dave thanked me and I went back to my own theatre. When I went into recovery an hour later, he recognised me from when I'd asked Frank to see him and he gave me the thumbs up. He stayed in hospital overnight and went home the following day. We did a variety of operations, cleft lips and palates, congenital deformities of ears, hands and feet and revision of burn scars.

Sara was an anaesthetist from Frank's hospital in Shavertown. I was called into her theatre where she was having trouble trying to intubate a boy of eighteen months. He was very small for his age, and clearly, from his appearance, had some sort of congenital syndrome. She'd been trying for some time to intubate him. She asked me to have a look and I was gently trying to gain a view of his cords when Dave appeared, followed by some of the Ecuadorian doctors. Sara insisted she wanted to have another attempt and almost snatched the laryngoscope off me.

In a situation like this the most important thing to me is to stay calm. If the patient is easy to ventilate, there is no rush. As long as they can be kept anaesthetised and oxygenated there is no real urgency and it is easy to forget this and this was exactly what I now saw was happening. To me, her attempts were very rough and forceful, as were Dave's and their sense of urgency, to me, was unnecessary.

I was fairly sure that they were causing trauma to the delicate lining of the upper airway close to the cords. If this leads to bleeding or swelling, intubation becomes even more difficult. Persistent attempts at intubation have led to deaths from upper airway obstruction. I asked how long she had been trying to intubate before I'd arrived. Twenty minutes. I said that they needed to stop. No one took any notice.

Sara was about to try again when I announced it was over.

'I'm sorry, but this needs to stop now. The whole situation is out of control and if you carry on you are going to kill him. It's not a competition to see who manages to get the tube in.' One of the local doctors, an anaesthetist, indicated he wanted to try too but I shook my head.

'It's over, wake him up.'

Frank wasn't happy, but I told him I didn't care. I was by far the most experienced anaesthetist there and I told him it wasn't his place to tell me they should carry on trying to intubate and put a child's life at risk. He was a surgeon not an anaesthetist. I told him if he wanted me to, I'd explain what had happened to the parents. There'd be other missions after ours and we could warn them so their own anaesthetists would be better prepared than we had been. He walked out, clearly still not happy. I waited until the toddler was starting to wake up before I went to start my next case.

At the end of the mission, we had a five-hour coach ride back to Guayaquil. I said goodbye to all but two the following morning, who like me had decided to have a couple of days to explore Guayaquil. One of them, a scrub nurse, was due to meet a friend the following afternoon from the US and the pair were then going to fly to Galapagos for a cruise around the islands.

I returned the following year, this time with my wife. It was a better mission in many ways, with no real issues or complications. In London we'd had a couple of nights relaxing before the long flight. She'd bought a cheap holdall, filling it with cuddly toys, clothes, crayons and colouring books for the children.

Coincidentally, the last day of work that week was our wedding anniversary and we celebrated with the rest of the team both occasions in a restaurant close to the hotel. Two days later, after the others had all set off for home, we flew to Galapagos for a four-night cruise around the islands on a private yacht.

If In Doubt

We saw giant turtles; I went snorkelling with Galapagos penguins and watched a flock of blue-footed booby birds as they flew overhead looking for a shoal of fish then diving like spears into the sea trying to catch them. We stepped over hundreds of black marine iguanas as we made our way along the beaches.

It was one of the most incredible experiences of my life. The yacht had only fourteen passengers and seven crew. We'd sail during the night, waking up at a different island each morning. It really was a once-in-a-lifetime adventure.

The following year was to me the best of all, although I was very concerned on the first morning at breakfast to find that apart from me there was only one anaesthetist from Florida, Ben, and he was relatively inexperienced in paediatric anaesthesia. There were meant to be two others, but they had dropped out at the last minute and Frank had thought seriously about cancelling the trip. The hospital was very keen that we came and had promised that two of their own anaesthetists would help whenever they could. There were two plastic surgeons and a Canadian orthopaedic surgeon who specialised in corrective surgery for congenital conditions affecting bones and tendons in the leg in children. He was one of the best surgeons I have ever worked with in my whole career.

There was one very difficult patient. She was sixteen and was listed to have a microtia operation. This was essentially an operation to create a new ear. Some children had been born with only a few pieces of skin and cartilage where the ear should have been but no recognisable external ear. This particular girl had an asymmetrical face too due to Goldenhar Syndrome. These patients were known to be in some cases extremely difficult to intubate.

I was unable to see any identifiable part of the airway around her larynx when I looked using the laryngoscope. I was about to wake her up and abandon her operation when Ben appeared. Frank said there was a video laryngoscope available. I'd not had much experience with this but Ben said he had used it a lot. He managed after a few minutes to intubate, but I had to keep reminding him to be as gentle as possible as again I felt he was being too forceful. He passed a very small tube into the airway and we confirmed it was in the right place and he left.

After intubation a seal is created by syringing air into a cuff around the tube. If this is not done some of the gas leaks back around the tube instead of going into the lungs making it difficult or impossible to ventilate. The seal also stops any blood or regurgitated fluid from contaminating the lungs. I checked for a leak and found that there wasn't one.

There was no air in the cuff but to me it was very worrying that there was also no leak. This meant that the small tube, which he'd pushed in using a lot of force in spite of me telling him to be gentle, was tightly wedged in the trachea. I was concerned that if the procedure took a long time, the effect of the tube pressing hard against the lining of the airway including the vocal cords for this time might cause it to swell once it was removed and cause potentially serious upper airway obstruction. In retrospect, there is no question that I should have abandoned the procedure at that point. Instead, I removed the tube and tried a laryngeal mask. The airway seemed perfect, so we proceeded with the surgery. It was a mistake.

After about two hours, small signs of airway obstruction started to develop. I told Frank I was becoming concerned but we were by now in the middle of the operation. At the end her oxygen saturation dropped. I was fairly certain that she had developed small patchy areas of lung collapse, or atelectasis, and had also probably aspirated some regurgitated fluid from her stomach which might have passed into her lungs.

I felt the essential thing was to get her awake as quickly as possible and ask her to deep-breathe and cough. I sat her up and also gave IV steroids and a nebuliser to try to open up the small airways.

The two anaesthetists who worked in the hospital told me that this type of patient could be very difficult to anaesthetise. They'd both seen situations where an emergency tracheostomy had been required to save the patient's life.

Fortunately, over the next hour or so she improved and within a few hours she didn't require additional oxygen and was breathing normally. She went home the following day, much to my relief.

At the end of this mission, my wife and I stayed on for a few days. A guide took us on a whole day trip in his jeep to see monkeys in the wild, incredible birds, amazing scenery and a visit to a cocoa plantation where we learnt how the beans were grown and we each made our own chocolate.

In 2017 I flew to General Santos in the Philippines to join a team with Operation Smile.

This charity started in 1982 and teams had carried out surgery for cleft lip and cleft palate repair in hundreds of thousands of children. It was to be by far the best week of my whole anaesthetic career. It is estimated a child is born with one of these conditions every three minutes. The website describes how '...many can't get access to surgery because it is too costly, too far away or too specialised. After-care is provided afterwards and depends on each child's needs, dentistry, speech therapy or psychotherapy…'

I had to take four flights to get there: Isle of Man to Gatwick, London to Dubai, Dubai to Manila and Manila to General Santos.

The thing that struck me was that the whole week was extremely well organised and safety was the main concern. First there was a team building day, a visit to a beautiful private beach by boat where we sunbathed, snorkelled and had a barbeque. That evening, back in General Santos, there was a meal and afterwards each team, with its leader, met and introduced themselves to each other. We discussed how the week would go and the type of general anaesthetic we'd give. There were seven other anaesthetists and there were to be six operating tables, three per theatre. I was a little worried that because this was my first mission with Operation Smile, I might have to just work alongside another anaesthetist for some of the time. I'd travelled a long way and wanted to do as much work on my own as I could, to give me the satisfaction I wanted.

Sunday was screening day. This took place in a large hall in a shopping centre. We arrived around 7.30 am to set it up, in readiness for the arrival of the children. There were to be a number of stations through which the potential patients would rotate. When we arrived there were no patients, but within an hour or so there were one hundred and seventy children and their parents. Seats had been set out in rows and they patiently awaited their turn. First their personal details would be taken and then they would be weighed, blood pressure and oxygen saturation would be measured and documented.

The surgeons would see all the children to ensure they could perform the necessary procedure then we would see them and assess their fitness for surgery. A paediatrician was at our station, on the lookout for anything we might miss, nipping in and out, listening to hearts and chests, ordering bloods in addition to the standard screening tests. Next the dentist and speech therapists would also make their own assessments.

At the end of a long day operating lists were displayed so that the parents would know when their child would be admitted to hospital and instructions on pre-operative fasting were explained to them. After assessment, every child had to go to the hospital to have blood taken for haemoglobin and electrolytes and any other investigations felt to be necessary such as a chest X-ray or ECG. To me, the overriding principle was one of safety, ensuring that the children were as fit as they could be in order to minimise any risk to them during and after surgery.

If In Doubt

    Looking back, this was something that had been missing in Ecuador, although I am as much to blame as anyone else for not realising it at the time. While the screening continued into the late afternoon, one of the other anaesthetists, Gavin, from Texas, had gone to the hospital to start with others to prepare the anaesthetic equipment in the two operating theatres.

The routine was for us to have breakfast from 6am and then there would be a meeting at 6.30 in the restaurant, with the coordinator giving an update on how things were going, how many patients we'd treated, any issues, where the meal that night would be and so on. There would then be a twenty-minute bus journey to the hospital. The team leader was planning to get me to work doubled up for a day or so before I would be allowed to work on my own, but Gavin from Texas was having none of it.

'That's Keith's table,' he said, 'I'm right here next to him if he needs anything, but he won't.' That was that. Sorted.

There were three tables in the theatre. An area in the corner was where the scrub nurse prepared and set out the instruments. The rule was that at the start of every anaesthetic two anaesthetists had to be present. The child, with their mother, would be checked by the anaesthetist or a nurse, then taken into the theatre. It struck me how the child's mother never cried or seemed in any way worried, in many cases there was no kiss as they handed over their child.

The trust that the mothers had in us was humbling to me. The younger ones were carried, but the older ones walked in, hand in hand with an anaesthetist. We'd walk past the other two tables, where operations were in progress and some would have a sly peek, craning their necks to try to see a little more. Very few became upset or cried. Most would be anaesthetised by gas through a face mask and once anaesthetised the other anaesthetist would insert an IV cannula and attach IV fluid. After intubation and having established that the airway had been secured, the other anaesthetist would leave.

If In Doubt

There were charts displayed on boards with algorithms for various anaesthetic events: anaphylaxis, a serious reaction to a drug, cardiac arrest and so on. To me, the whole atmosphere oozed safety. At home, I might be the only anaesthetist in the hospital in the middle of the night with a high-risk patient needing emergency surgery and if anything went wrong and I needed assistance, I knew it would be maybe thirty minutes before it would come. This was the opposite in a way; it was elective surgery and there would be seven other anaesthetists literally next to me throughout the entire anaesthetic. Three or four anaesthetists in one theatre and three or four next door.

There were careful checks at every stage and excellent surgeons from the Philippines, Japan, Canada and the US. A paediatrician worked in the recovery ward nearby with the recovery nurses. It was extremely rewarding to see a child with a cleft lip, or even worse bilateral cleft, come for surgery and an hour or so later leave with a perfect face. I almost felt it would have been worth travelling all that way even for one day just to be able to see the faces of the children and their parents after surgery. They'd go to the recovery room for an hour or so after their operation then they all would stay overnight with a parent in a large room with around fifty camp beds. An intensive care paediatrician from England was in charge of this room. Two nurses on the team stayed with them all through the night. During the entire week, there were no serious pain or airway issues. Each night we'd have a meal together before heading back to the hotel and the whole experience was well-organised, sometimes sad, but funny at times too, and most certainly rewarding. The rest of the team were incredible.

It had been a week I'd never forget, probably the best of my whole thirty-seven-year career. A big regret for me is that I didn't do more of this sort of work. Covid19 would put paid to my plans for that. All such missions had to stop until the pandemic was under control and by then I'd be retired.

CHAPTER 11

Hope

One of the most difficult things I have found during my career is deciding what to say to patients who are very ill and their relatives, and how to say it. Many doctors feel that when difficult decisions are being made about a patient who may die and the outlook seems poor, they should paint the worst possible picture.

I've heard this expression many times. The doctor may feel that if they say they are expecting the patient will not do well and might even die and then they do die, the relatives won't be too surprised and won't have any cause for complaint as that was what they were expecting anyway. If, on the other hand, the patient eventually made a good recovery, the expectation is that the relatives might think the doctor and nurses have done a fantastic job. So in creating this feeling of pessimism, the doctors and nurses might feel they have a win-win situation.

This may sound like a reasonable approach on the face of it, but I have always felt it is not really acceptable in some cases, perhaps in any cases. I've thought about this a lot over the years and I have come to the conclusion that it isn't right unless the doctor saying it honestly believes it is true. Leading on from this, it is clear that if the doctor honestly feels that there is a reasonable chance that the patient could make a good recovery, the family deserves to be told this too with as equal importance as the bad news that they'd been given.

There are no guarantees in medicine, doctors are relying on their knowledge and experience in advising patients and their loved ones. But my own feeling is that if it is felt that there is hope and the possibility of a good recovery, they should be told this. I think this hope is essential for the family in helping them to deal with the situation they find themselves in. Honesty and hope might help them deal with the situation. Weeks or months of misery and worry for the relatives because of a very poor prognosis may be unfounded and the patient might make a good recovery.

To be in a position to be able to walk this very fine line between optimism and pessimism when it comes to talking to a patient or their relatives, of course, the doctor has to have the experience to back it up. There is no place for just guessing, but I do feel a 'gut feeling' is important and I often say this when discussing possible outcomes. Backed up by involvement with patients in similar situations, knowledge and general experience gained over many years, a gut feeling, to me anyway, has an important role in the way information is given to patients and their family. This applies to nurses as well as doctors.

Mike was a forty-seven-year-old man who'd crashed his motorbike into a tree after losing control at high speed. He was conscious at the scene and when he was brought into the A&E department, but it was clear that he had serious leg and chest injuries. A conscious patient is a very reassuring sign. Whatever may be wrong with them, it at least allows staff to know the brain has probably not had a serious injury. Even if there are no other injuries, a severe brain injury can easily kill a patient. The initial assessment of any patient follows the same principle. A rapid primary assessment is the first priority.

This is an 'A to E' assessment of airway, breathing, circulation, disability and exposure. In the primary assessment, if a patient is conscious and talking, this reassures medical and nursing staff that the airway is open, he or she is breathing and also must have a reasonable circulation as blood is being carried to the brain. The reason 'airway' comes first is not simply that A is the first letter of the alphabet and B second. Airway compromise will kill a patient before a breathing problem.

If In Doubt

A quick assessment of airway and breathing takes place. If necessary, the airway is opened and oxygen given via a face mask. The chest is examined, looking at the pattern of breathing for symmetry of chest movement, listening with a stethoscope. A chest X-ray might be indicated. In 'C', cool hands and feet might indicate inadequate circulation, shock, perhaps from blood loss. The pulse, its rate and character, blood pressure, neck vein filling and heart are examined. The abdomen too is examined, looking for signs that there may be bleeding there. I've always found assessment here to be very difficult. Ultrasound scanning can help but urgent CT scanning is the main investigation now in assessing intra-abdominal injuries and haemorrhage.

Massive blood loss can also occur behind it, so there is no free blood sloshing around, it's all in the tissues contained behind the peritoneum, making it even harder to detect. This is termed retroperitoneal bleeding. A fractured pelvis often causes this type of haemorrhage. 'On the floor and four more,' is a term often used to remind a doctor of the likely sites of massive blood loss. On the floor means at the scene of an accident. If a large amount is actually seen it is clear there has been a lot of blood loss externally. Paramedics often photograph the scene so the doctors in the hospital can get an idea of the mechanism of the injuries and also an idea of the amount of blood lost there. The other four are bleeding into the chest cavity, intra-abdominal, retroperitoneal and from a fractured femur, thigh bone or, worse still, two fractured femurs. The femur is the largest bone in the body and a lot of blood, maybe one and a half litres or more, can be lost in the tissues around the fracture site. The average circulating blood volume for an adult is around five litres, so bilateral femur fractures can lead to a loss of around three litres, approximately 60% of the total blood in the body.

'D' stands for disability and means neurological disability. The main thing to note here is the conscious level and this is measured using a scoring system which involves looking at eye opening, motor function, if there is movement in the limbs, and the verbal response which can range from normal conversation to a patient making no sounds at all. The Glasgow Coma Score is used to determine the level of consciousness. 'E' is exposure, removing clothing and examining the whole external part of the body. After this initial assessment decisions are made about treatment and this is then started. Any life-threatening injuries are dealt with as they are found.

Mike complained of pain in his chest and multiple rib fractures were seen on his chest X-ray. There was patchy shadowing suggestive of contusion, or bruising, of both lungs and a haemothorax, blood in the chest cavity outside the lung itself. This usually requires a chest drain to allow the blood to escape into a large bottle. There was bruising and abrasions over the left side of his abdomen, which was distended and tense. It was obvious from the deformity of his left thigh that Mike had a fracture of the femur. His lower leg was cold and mottled and no pulses could be felt suggesting a vascular injury caused by the sharp bone fragments at the fracture site. Blood was ordered and he was taken to theatre after a CT scan revealed a ruptured spleen with a large amount of blood in the abdomen.

A general surgeon removed the spleen and another scan showed no blood flow to the leg below the fracture. The femur was nailed by an orthopaedic surgeon and a graft inserted by the vascular surgeon to restore the blood flow. It is essential to repair the artery as soon as possible because the leg muscle cells can die after a few hours and amputation may then become necessary. At the end of an eight-hour operation his respiratory function had worsened, so he was needing 70% oxygen to ensure enough was getting through his damaged lungs and into the blood.

The chemical reaction within the cells needed to create the energy required to keep the cells alive needs oxygen. If deprived of it they can die; some, like brain cells, more quickly than others. It was clear that he wouldn't be able to breathe on his own, so he was kept anaesthetised on a ventilator in ICU after the operation. Over the next two weeks, things went from bad to worse. His lower left leg, the muscles damaged by the long period without blood, swelled causing compartment syndrome.

The groups of muscles are contained in 'compartments' enclosed by tough tissue called fascia. If the muscles swell after injury the pressure within the compartment rises and blood flow in the tiny capillaries carrying blood and oxygen to the cells is reduced or may stop completely. The treatment for this is an urgent fasciotomy where the surgeon makes an incision through the skin down to the fascia. An incision in that too leaves it open to release the pressure within the swollen and tense muscle. Blood flow is restored. He had slowly developed multiple organ failure. He had respiratory failure from severe contusion and also now infection and was still on the ventilator.

His kidneys had failed and he was receiving renal support, or being dialysed. He also had liver failure and this had affected the way in which his blood was clotting so that his wounds were oozing. There is a very high mortality rate with this condition, which rises as the number of organs failing increases. The survival rates have probably not improved from what they were thirty or forty years ago.

When renal support is given blood is taken out of the body and passed through a 'filter' which takes out impurities and returns it back into the body. To prevent the blood clotting in the lines, an anticoagulant, IV Heparin is given during dialysis. In Mike's case this had led to bleeding from the fasciotomy wound from multiple sites and he was requiring multiple transfusions of blood to replace this. This had been going on for several days.

I was on call one evening and went to the ICU. I immediately saw how bad things had now become. The nurses had been putting dressings over the wound and pressing firmly on them to try to slow down the steady flow of blood, but this was clearly not working. His condition was so awful that some of my colleagues were wondering if we should not simply accept that he was going to die. The wound had also become infected and bacteria had grown from his blood cultures. He had septicaemic shock requiring drugs like adrenaline to support his circulation and so had four organ failures: lung, kidney, liver and circulation. The mortality rate would probably be around 80-90%, perhaps even higher. As I removed the dressing on the thigh wound and saw the bleeding points, I had an idea.

Diathermy is used in the operating theatre to burn or cauterise small bleeding vessels to seal them. I wheeled the machine round to the ICU and tried to contact a surgeon and ask if they would try to carry out diathermy on the bleeding. The two on-call surgeons were in theatre and would be several hours but sent back a message saying I could try it myself and suggested the settings on the machine. I spent about an hour using diathermy to stop bleeding from the tiny bleeding points.

The infusion of Heparin, which had been stopped in an attempt to reduce the bleeding, despite the risk of blood clotting in the lines and his dialysis having to stop again, was re-started. There was no further bleeding and a colleague walked into the unit at this point.

'I know it looks really bad,' I said, 'but for some reason, I just think he will make a full recovery.'

Lungs, kidneys and liver can all heal and recover completely and my gut feeling here was that this would happen. I think he was surprised as by then I knew I was developing a reputation for being over-pessimistic in general with some intensive care patients. If it appeared completely hopeless, I couldn't stop myself from telling nurses, doctors and relatives just that. On the other hand, if I felt there was hope, even if colleagues disagreed, I would tell them that too and I personally felt strongly that with this patient we needed to press on and hope things came right. In Mike's case they did. About four weeks later he left the ICU and eventually made his way home to Ireland. He sent a letter about five months later to say he was pretty much back to his normal self and back to work.

A fifteen-year-old boy, Rory, was admitted to the ICU feeling generally unwell and was suspected of having sepsis. In this condition, usually caused by bacteria, the body's own defences against an infection, the immune system, for an unknown reason attacks organs and can cause them to fail and can lead to death in severe cases.

He'd complained of headaches and generalised aches and pains and had vomited several times. Earlier that day he'd become drowsy on the ward and the doctors there were concerned that if his conscious level worsened, he would not be able to maintain it and might need to have a tube inserted in order to protect it if he vomited again.

The suspected diagnosis was meningitis and tests were carried out in an attempt to identify the source of the infection. After a few days a bacteria was grown from blood cultures and was found to be resistant to the IV antibiotic he'd been receiving since admission so this was changed. His conscious level had worsened and he'd been placed on a ventilator. A CT scan looked normal and an MRI scan was requested.

For this procedure there must be no metal anywhere in the scan room and special MRI-compatible anaesthetic machines and monitoring equipment are required. We didn't have this at our hospital at that time so I kept him anaesthetised but took him off the ventilator in ICU and watched his breathing for about fifteen minutes to assess whether I felt he would be safe to have the scan. Although his breathing rate was fast, I knew he'd not come to any harm for the time it would take, around thirty minutes, as long as he had adequate oxygen throughout the procedure.

I went into the scanner with him as we had no monitoring apart from me watching his breathing, his colour and feeling his pulse.

After it was completed, I was shown the brain scan by the radiologist. The brain contained multiple abscesses of varying size scattered throughout and these were the cause of his symptoms including the decreased conscious level. I took him back to the ICU and went with a nurse to talk to his parents in the visitor's room. They were devastated and as this condition is quite rare I didn't feel in a position to speculate on the likely outcome and the chances of a full recovery. His mother cried uncontrollably.

After a few minutes I asked if they would mind if I left them with the nurse for about ten minutes but would be back soon. I stepped into the corridor outside the ICU and asked to be put through to the Regional Neurosurgical Centre at Walton Hospital in Liverpool. I asked the switchboard operator if I could speak to a consultant neurosurgeon and I described Rory's condition to him. I described the MRI scan appearance and asked if he might be able to give me an idea of the likely outcome. I said his parents were really upset and I wanted to get as much information as possible before I spoke to them again. He said things were serious, but he also felt that treatment with the correct intravenous antibiotic, which he was now receiving, could still lead to a full recovery. He'd seen similar situations before. There was no place for surgery; the treatment was a six-week course of IV antibiotics. I told his parents this news and they visibly became less upset almost immediately.

'He said he wouldn't be surprised if he makes a full recovery, without any long-term neurological deficit,' I told them.

'He's optimistic.'

A few days later, Rory was found to have a heart murmur. Combined with positive blood cultures and the multiple brain abscesses, it became clear that the diagnosis was infective endocarditis, a bacterial infection of the heart valves. The treatment for this was six weeks of intravenous antibiotics.

Although it was a long journey Rory made a full recovery but he did require a period of rehabilitation for his brain injury after being in the ICU for four weeks and the paediatric ward for another six weeks. Apart from a gut feeling I think it is important in this type of situation to go straight to the top and ask a consultant who specialises in the particular condition we need to know more about. This sort of optimism is almost infectious – if I hadn't rung the surgeon, it might have meant more weeks of uncertainty, more sleepless nights and more stress for his parents. The whole atmosphere in the ICU seemed to change from all doom and gloom to upbeat. The MRI scan had looked so bad it was hard to believe that the patient could again have a normal brain, whatever treatment he was given. With an opinion like this though, from a very experienced and well–respected neurosurgeon, which took only a few minutes to obtain, the mood changed dramatically. In this sort of difficult situation I've felt this approach is a good one for the relatives, doctors and nurses.

Brian was admitted to the ICU with respiratory, renal and liver failure and signs of infection. He was thirty-one, a gardener and had been working in a garden adjacent to a river for the previous few months. He was deeply jaundiced, a yellow discoloration of the skin and the whites of the eyes, the sclera, caused by high blood levels of bilirubin in the blood due to liver failure. Leptospirosis. This is a rare bacterial infection caused by a bacteria called Leptospira which is excreted in the urine of animals, often rats. It is more common in tropical climates and about ninety percent of cases are mild, not requiring hospital admission. For some, though, the illness can be severe and can result in death. It was clear that he was in this ten percent. Renal support, dialysis, was started and his breathing became more laboured. He was placed on a ventilator after four days in the ICU.

He had three organ system failures but over the next two days he required circulatory support. One of the effects of some of the chemicals released into the blood during severe infection is for the blood vessels to dilate, or get wider.

Blood pools in these dilated veins and not as much blood returns to the heart after picking up oxygen in the lungs then being pumped around the body by the heart. This leads to a drop in blood pressure and poor oxygen delivery to the tissues, the condition called shock. Intravenous fluids were given and a drug which constricts and squeezes the dilated blood vessels, Noradrenaline, was given by continuous IV infusion. Over the next two days his general condition worsened, and two colleagues had spoken to his partner and both told her they felt there was a good chance he might not survive. With three small children she was extremely upset.

I was on call one evening from five o'clock and went to see him as I'd not been involved in his care since his admission to ICU. He'd been very fit, a race walker, non-smoker with no illnesses. My gut feeling was that he'd make a good recovery. I went to introduce myself to his partner who was only about twenty-five and in tears, sitting alone in the visitors' room. I told her this condition was quite rare but I'd seen around five during the previous twelve years or so. All had been ill enough to need intensive care but all had made full recoveries. It was clear, I said that he was very ill but the fact he was very fit normally would help his recovery. I explained he was definitely on the right antibiotic; the bacteria had been shown to be sensitive to it and from the blood tests there was some evidence the drug was starting to have an effect. Again, my gut feeling was that he'd make a complete recovery and I explained this too although I told her I was fairly sure he might need a tracheostomy to help us to get him off the ventilator as there was no sign of his lung function recovering quickly.

She stopped crying and looked up, looking surprised, saying she'd been told the outlook was poor. One of my colleagues had told her he could well die. I explained I'd seen other patients with severe infections and multiple organ failure do well and honestly felt he would too although obviously I couldn't guarantee it. It took about five weeks for him to be well enough to leave the ICU but he eventually made a complete recovery and returned to work as a gardener.

Discussions with patients or, if they are unconscious, their relatives can be very difficult. Having several colleagues involved helps as a consensus can be arrived at, but even then there is often uncertainty. Every patient is different. Some may be very fit while others of the same age may, for example, be heavy smokers with associated chronic lung disease or ischaemic heart disease or both, which might make them less likely to be able to fight a severe illness. On the one hand the hope is, for the doctors and nurses, that we can give each the best possible chance of a good recovery. On the other hand though, we don't want the patient to suffer unnecessarily if it later becomes clear that the outcome will inevitably end in death. It can be difficult and I feel this will always be the case.

If a particular condition has been shown statistically to have a 99% mortality rate, how do we know that our patient isn't in the 1% tiny minority group? Of course we can't know. All we can do is use our experience, sometimes taking note of our 'gut feeling' and be honest. Involving others in decision making including sometimes speaking with those in other hospitals too is important.

I was first on call one night, meaning I had to live in the hospital all night and be available for anything that might happen – emergency surgery, trauma calls to A&E, pain issues on the wards, obstetric emergencies and so on. In the ICU I took the handover from a colleague who'd been covering it all day. He told me about Jim, a seventy-four-year-old man who was on a week's holiday on the island and had collapsed while walking along the promenade that morning. A relative suspected a cardiac arrest and had started chest compressions after a few minutes and the paramedics had arrived after about ten minutes, confirmed he had suffered a cardiac arrest and taken over CPR. Jim had suffered a cardiac arrest in the ambulance on the way into hospital and required a shock with a defibrillator to restart his heart. In A&E there had been two more episodes of VF, ventricular fibrillation, from which he was also successfully defibrillated. My colleague told me that he was clearly now in cardiac failure, on drugs to support his heart (inotropes) and had been sedated and ventilated.

He'd had a long discussion with Jim's wife and two sons and had told them that he felt the outlook was so poor that in his opinion the best way forward would be to withdraw support and allow him to die peacefully. He felt the likelihood of his brain being normal was very small after the cardiac arrest and delay in him receiving CPR with oxygen by the paramedics. The ECG showed a large myocardial infarction, or heart attack, and this had caused his heart to fail. He added some more family wanted to see him before we did and were coming in around 10pm and then we were stopping all treatment and he was expected to die very quickly.

I asked what his pupils were doing, and my colleague admitted he didn't know. If these are not reacting to light or unequal and reacting only sluggishly this can suggest a hypoxic brain injury, although some of these signs are unreliable. This type of injury can also lead to seizures, a very worrying sign indeed after an out-of-hospital cardiac arrest, almost always indicating a serious brain injury. There'd been no seizures so far. After he went off duty the nursing staff and his family were prepared for withdrawal of treatment a little later that evening.

I went to examine him after my consultant colleague had left. He was anaesthetised and on a ventilator, with a high dose of inotropic drugs. He was on 60% oxygen which indicated likely lung congestion due to heart failure, although the chest X-ray showed only mild failure and his chest sounded clear. Urine output was poor suggesting he may also be developing renal failure but the pupils reacted normally. I had another 'gut feeling' moment.

I spoke to the nurse looking after him for the night who was very experienced, and she also felt we should withdraw soon. I wasn't so sure and waited to speak to his family. I asked them about his exercise tolerance – how much physical exertion he was capable of and his quality of life. He could walk slowly around a quarter of a mile without stopping and could walk upstairs without stopping, although again taking his time. He'd been a heavy smoker but had stopped five years earlier after a heart attack. He went to the pub several nights a week and pottered about in his greenhouse. I told them it did appear that the outlook wasn't good, but I felt a little uncomfortable about withdrawing so quickly. They looked surprised.

'We were told he would definitely die this evening,' his son said.

This sort of situation is difficult, where two doctors disagree and I explained this. I explained that I'd spoken to my colleague and his opinion was that it was completely hopeless. I felt there was still hope and there would be no harm in carrying on, at least overnight. Again, it was only a gut feeling but I did say that I wouldn't be surprised if he woke up if we got to the stage where we could safely do that to assess his neurological function. They were aware that there was a DNAR so if he suffered another cardiac arrest he wasn't going to be resuscitated.

During the night I gave some boluses of fluid and some drugs to help treat his cardiac failure and slowly reduced the sedation. When my shift ended at 8am his oxygen requirement was only 30%, suggesting his failure was less, urine output had picked up and he was starting to cough on the tube. There had been no abnormal posturing or seizures which would probably have indicated a brain injury. At the handover I said I felt that all the sedation should be stopped and he should be extubated and assessed neurologically. My feeling was that he would easily be able to breathe on his own and would slowly wake up. This is what happened and the following day he was starting to say a few words although still drowsy.

Three days later he was eating and drinking, requiring only nasal oxygen and he was transferred to the CCU. His family were delighted but knew he might at any moment have another cardiac arrest. My feeling was that plans should be made to get him back home to Wales at that point but the cardiologist was reluctant to do this. Unfortunately, after a week or so, when he had been making good progress, he suffered another arrest. Resuscitation was not carried out and he died.

His family sent a lovely card thanking me. It is always very difficult to know the best way forward in such a situation. As long as the patient doesn't suffer I feel continuing to give them a chance is reasonable if anyone in the team feels strongly that this is appropriate. I felt here that there was a possibility he might slowly recover although when I first became involved a decision had already been made to withdraw. Continuing with support for a while can always be later changed to withdrawal and acceptance that death is inevitable.

Changing the plan isn't possible though when a decision to withdraw is made and death follows quickly; there is no coming back from that.

CHAPTER 12

Dilemmas

For a doctor there are certain taboos and breaking these can lead to all kinds of problems, some with serious consequences. The GMC has a code of practice and if a doctor steps outside of this there might be repercussions. The ultimate sanction is being struck off the medical register, signalling the end of a career. For example, starting a relationship with a patient, being involved in a criminal act or an accusation of racism can all lead to serious trouble for any doctor.

One aspect of my own work as a consultant in the only hospital on the island, has been the dilemma when a close family member needs advice or treatment, maybe surgery or admission to the ICU. At times this has led to me having to think carefully and balance the need for their care and how that care is given against my own opinions or involvement.

There is no law which prohibits a doctor treating his own family, The GMC, however, would certainly frown on this in most cases on ethical grounds. Overstepping the mark could potentially lead me into dangerous territory. The same applies to many doctors on the Isle of Man or any small island with only one hospital. Ideally in a situation like this all decisions and care should be passed on to a colleague. On a small island with a relatively small number of colleagues this is not always possible.

John, a consultant anaesthetist friend, asked me if I was on the island for the following two weeks as his wife was due to have their first child. He asked if I could look after her if necessary, if she needed an epidural or a caesarean section. I told him I'd be pleased to do this and wasn't planning any trips off island. For any doctor it is almost an honour to be asked by a colleague if you will look after either them or a family member. For me that usually meant anaesthetising them. As a little perk, doctors, often nurses too, sometimes make a request like this.

I once told a fairly junior anaesthetist he had a VIP on his operating list the following day – my middle daughter. I could have asked any of my consultant colleagues to anaesthetise her. I think one or two of them were surprised when I didn't do this. After her operation he came to thank me for trusting him. I told him if I didn't feel he was good enough he wouldn't be allowed to anaesthetise any patient. If I and my other consultant colleagues allowed him to be working unsupervised at night as the only anaesthetist in the hospital, we had to believe he was capable.

This was in the days before mobile phones. I carried my bleep around every day when in the hospital for the next few weeks. I'd also told the switchboard they could ring my house phone at any time if for some reason the bleep wasn't answered. A week later, about nine o'clock on a Saturday morning, I went into the hospital to see some patients I'd anaesthetised the previous day and some in the ICU I'd been looking after. I wasn't on call that weekend – John himself was. As I was driving in I realised I'd left my bleep at home.

Walking through the main entrance past the switchboard, one of the operators called to me, 'They need you urgently in the Jane.'

The obstetric unit at the island's hospital is named the Jane Crookall Maternity Unit, known to all as the Jane. One of the consultant obstetricians was going into the changing rooms and he spotted me. 'Have you heard what's happened?' he said, shaking his head. 'The shit's hit the fan.'

I told him I knew nothing but guessed it might have something to do with John's wife. He told me she'd gone into early labour a few hours previously. The midwives had found the baby to be in a breech position, bottom first, the head high in the uterus. There are risks to the baby in allowing the mother to continue in labour with a breech, so a caesarean section is now felt to be the preferred method of delivering the baby.

There is, however, a possible way of avoiding a caesarean. It is sometimes possible to turn the baby around by manoeuvring it through the abdominal wall. This procedure is called an external cephalic version, or ECV. The risk is that the placenta can be pulled away from the wall of the uterus and the blood supply to the fetus via the umbilical cord can suddenly be compromised. This results in fetal distress, seen by changes on the CTG, or cardiotocography monitor. This machine continuously monitors contractions and the changes in heart rate accompanying them. About one in two hundred require an immediate section.

There is a saying in medicine that if things are going to go wrong, they will go wrong with a doctor or a nurse as the patient. Or a close relative of a doctor or nurse. It had certainly gone badly wrong here. During the ECV there'd been a dramatic fall in heart rate, and it was suspected that there was severe fetal compromise. An urgent caesarean section was required. I quickly changed and went into the anaesthetic room.

John was drawing up drugs, getting ready to anaesthetise her himself if they couldn't find me.

'Thank God you're here!' he said. 'I was getting worried I'd have to do it myself.'

There'd be no time for him to start ringing around trying to find another colleague to come in. The other anaesthetist on call with him that day was in theatre with an elderly lady having surgery for her fractured hip. I gave John's wife a spinal anaesthetic and their daughter was born about fifteen minutes later and was fine after a brief period of resuscitation. There'd been the potential for a very bad scenario and we both knew it but we never talked about it later. It was too awful to even think about.

If John had gone ahead with a spinal and it was unsuccessful, which can happen, she'd have needed a general anaesthetic. It was known the baby had signs of fetal distress and might well need prolonged resuscitation. Often the paediatrician involved would request the help of the anaesthetist. So, he might have found himself in a situation where he had to look after his wife, who he had just anaesthetised while at the same time having to also resuscitate his own baby.

We never mentioned any of this, but both knew this could have so easily been a reality. It had been a close shave. He would never have got himself in any trouble with the GMC as the situation he could have found himself in was unforeseen. It would be obvious to anyone that he was acting to save the life of his own baby, and the only way he might have been able to do that would have been by anaesthetising his own wife as quickly as possible.

Early pregnancy miscarriages are relatively common; around one in four to five end this way. Like many others, I know from personal experience how upsetting this can be. Throughout my long career I must have anaesthetised many hundreds of patients who needed surgical removal of 'retained products of conception.' This terribly tragic phrase refers to when parts of the fetus or placenta are not expelled from the uterus during the miscarriage. If not removed they can cause pain and bleeding and may become infected. The operation for these – Evacuation of Retained Products of Conception (ERPC), now termed Surgical Management of Miscarriage (SMM), is usually, and quite understandably, a distressing experience for the patient.

One of the saddest things I ever had to deal with during my career, and I always felt the same, was when it was necessary to be involved in the care of a patient who had had late intrauterine fetal death, or IUFD. This is when a baby is carried almost to full term with all the excitement

If In Doubt

that brings as preparations are made in anticipation of the new arrival.

The mother would probably have reported that recently there'd been no movement from the fetus. The midwife would have carried out a scan and confirmed that the baby had died.

To be told this, sometimes only a few days before your child is due to be born, must be heart-breaking for everyone involved, but especially the mother.

In the past, these patients were treated expectantly. This meant they were forced to wait until labour started naturally and the baby would usually be born via a normal vaginal delivery. In some cases, this meant the mother would have to carry the dead baby for several weeks. Now, in order to prevent this, labour is usually induced soon after the diagnosis has been made.

My own involvement with these patients would begin when a midwife asked if I might consider an epidural for pain relief. Although there are other forms of analgesia during labour, the most effective, if it works well, is undoubtedly an epidural. Often the patient has no pain at all during the rest of the labour once an epidural starts to work.

As I'm sure all anaesthetists do, I have always tried to ensure the epidural is as effective as possible with all obstetric patients – but especially in these ones during what must be an incredibly traumatic experience. I've always felt that the very least I could do was to try to give them, at least physically, as pain-free a labour as possible. I'd always tell the midwife to call me for anything at all during the labour, so I could top up the epidural and give an extra dose of local anaesthetic if required. If the epidural wasn't particularly effective, as can sometimes happen, I'd take it out and insert another one.

My oldest daughter developed mild pre-eclampsia towards the end of her first pregnancy nine years ago. Pre-eclampsia is a disorder of pregnancy that affects approximately one in twenty pregnant women. It usually occurs after thirty-two weeks – normal duration of pregnancy is about forty weeks. Some patients have no symptoms, only high blood pressure and protein in their urine. The exact cause of the condition remains unknown, but it is thought to result from an abnormal placenta. The placenta connects the unborn baby to the mother via the umbilical cord and is attached to the inside of the uterus. Oxygen and nutrients, necessary for the growth and survival of the fetus, pass from the mother's blood into the baby's, via the placenta and umbilical cord. Abnormal development of the placenta leads to poor blood flow, or perfusion. This is one of the potential causes of IUFD.

My daughter had been seen a couple of times in the clinic and a week before had been told by the consultant obstetrician that he wanted to see her again in a week or so and she'd get an appointment in the post. A week later she rang me one lunchtime. She hadn't received the appointment and was unsure what to do. I therefore told her I'd ring the obstetrician. I anaesthetised for his gynaecology list every Wednesday and I'd worked with him for about twelve years. He told me not to worry and suggested she see him at the start of his clinic, at 2pm that day. I told her this and I was in theatre that afternoon when she rang to tell me he wanted her to come into hospital overnight so she could have continuous CTG monitoring. He'd said she should go home, get some bits and pieces for the overnight stay and come back to the obstetric ward and she'd probably be able to go home in the morning. I saw her on my way home at about 6.30pm.

At around 3am the following morning the phone by the bed woke us. My daughter said they'd suddenly become concerned about the trace on the CTG monitor and she was going for an urgent caesarean section. My wife and I went into the hospital and as we arrived, I saw her briefly as she was about to have a spinal anaesthetic for the operation. For the next half an hour or so we waited anxiously at the desk in the labour ward, grateful when an ODP finally came out and said everything was fine and we'd be able to see her soon. She'd had a boy – our first grandchild. We heard that when he'd been born he'd needed resuscitation.

Often the trace would suggest fetal distress, meaning that the life of the baby was at risk. An urgent section would then be carried out, but the baby would sometimes come out screaming, clearly not in the least bit distressed. Here though, the trace had indicated there was a serious problem, and there had been.

We got home around 5.45am and, coincidentally, I was working that day with the obstetrician who had seen her in the clinic. He'd not been on call during the night, but he'd heard about the section and had seen the CTG trace.

'What was the trace like?' I asked as we were in the coffee room waiting to start the day's operating list.

He looked at me for a few seconds.

'Bloody awful,' he said.

If she hadn't rung me, if I hadn't rung him, if he'd said,

'Oh, the clinic is full this afternoon but not to worry, I'll see her in the morning.'

The realisation of what might have happened because my daughter hadn't received her appointment was so awful, I immediately blocked it from entering my thoughts. The obstetrician and I never spoke of it again, but the reality is that if she hadn't gone into the obstetric ward that afternoon her baby would almost certainly have died that night while she slept. The next morning, she might have noticed there were no movements, no more little kicks. As with many other scenarios I've seen during my career it was yet another reminder of the fragility of life. It can end before it has even started.

Maybe it was because I was so busy working, with so little time to think, but with our own children I don't think I worried about them so much. With my beautiful grandchildren though I worry about everything, I can't help it. My eldest grandson, the one whose birth I've just described, is a motorcycle trials rider and I watch him whenever I can. If I see a difficult section, I imagine the worst and a crash. Instinctively – I can't seem to stop myself – I move to the spot where he might fall, so I can at least try to catch him. My oldest granddaughter, his cousin, is a gymnast. As she somersaults and back-flips across the floor, flies between the asymmetric bars and – to me, the worst of all, performs her routine on the beam, I can sometimes hardly bear to watch. They have to follow their dreams. But I still worry about them.

My father-in-law, Jim, was a great mechanic. A tough, no-nonsense Manxman, he was proud of his family and all they had achieved, hard-working and very funny at times. Like his wife, June, he loved singing and I used to like nights out with them with my wife, when invariably they would do a duet, singing *True Love* to each other as they gazed lovingly into each other's eyes.

He suffered from chronic obstructive lung disease caused by many years of heavy smoking. Like millions of others before the dangers associated with passive smoking became known, my own dad included, he smoked in the house. June suffered from asthma. Her own mother had died during an asthma attack when June was a toddler.

During the first seven years or so that I knew Jim, I watched a steady deterioration in his health until the inevitable happened and he was admitted to hospital in 1990, during my first year as a consultant at Noble's Hospital, with a sudden worsening of his condition, an exacerbation of COPD. In spite of having frequent courses of antibiotics and bronchodilator drugs via a nebuliser to open up the constricted small airways in his lungs it was clear to me that he was going to end up in the ICU soon and might well not come out alive.

After a few days on a medical ward, he was transferred to the unit and his breathing was so bad he had to be anaesthetised, intubated and placed on a ventilator. My wife's two brothers and two sisters lived in London, and I rang them and explained the seriousness of the situation.

After a week or so he was taken off the ventilator and two days later, a Sunday, I was on call when he again deteriorated. In those days, the early 1990s, we had trainee anaesthetists in the anaesthetic department and I was on call with one who was only in their first few months of training, so he was very inexperienced. During the week there would have been three other consultant anaesthetists but being a weekend, I was basically on my own. I tried several drugs without success and it rapidly became clear that he needed to be anaesthetised and put back on the ventilator. I asked one of my colleagues if he would come in and help to get Jim back on the ventilator.

Although I knew my colleague couldn't really do any more than I could, I was uncomfortable with the fact he was my father-in-law, he was very ill and my wife and the rest of her family were obviously worried. More importantly, I also knew that even after the tube had been inserted into his trachea, he might be very difficult to ventilate. Even impossible. If that happened, I'd have a very serious situation to deal with and there was a possibility he could die. In some cases of severe asthma or COPD there could be such severe bronchospasm – constriction of the tiny airways in the lungs – that it was almost impossible to squeeze oxygen in.

Many years later I would see it for the first and only time in my anaesthetic career. On call one night, the phone rang just after midnight, and I was asked to attend A&E urgently. A twelve-year-old girl who suffered from asthma had developed sudden breathlessness. Her inhalers had been ineffective and by the time an ambulance arrived she'd collapsed, unconscious. The paramedics had struggled to ventilate her and she'd been intubated in A&E by my colleague but he had been unable to ventilate her. She was in cardiac arrest.

If In Doubt

I arrived several minutes after the call. Her parents stood a few yards from their daughter, watching the resuscitation. The first on-call anaesthetist, who stayed in the hospital all night, had intubated her. I took over trying to ventilate her. It was as if someone had placed a clamp over the tracheal tube –however hard the bag was squeezed, there was no chest movement at all. During my whole career, I'd never seen anything like this. I felt completely helpless; I could get no oxygen into her lungs via the tracheal tube. She was in asystole and was receiving chest compressions and intravenous adrenaline. The best way to get results from bronchodilator drugs is via a nebuliser, which produces minute droplets containing the drug and these pass into the small airways and act on receptors in cells lining the airway. In severe cases – and this was by far the worst asthma attack I had ever seen – the drug can't be given that way and the only way for it to be effective is through the intravenous route. Several drugs had been given this route and the adrenaline being given every four minutes for cardiac arrest is also an excellent bronchodilator, but all had been completely ineffective.

During an asthma attack or exacerbation of COPD, air passes into the lungs as it is sucked in by the increased effort of breathing. However, not as much passes out of the lungs on expiration. Listening with a stethoscope, an expiratory wheeze is heard –the whistling sound produced by air passing through the constricted airways. This leads to the lungs becoming over-distended, or hyper-inflated. The main muscle of breathing is the diaphragm. This becomes more and more flattened and stretched so that it eventually becomes ineffective. I tried a manoeuvre that is rarely required or used – manually compressing the chest, squeezing it to try and get some of the air out and allow it to deflate. By doing that we might be able to then squeeze some oxygen in.

If In Doubt

After a minute or so of this some chest movement became visible on inspiration and suddenly ECG complexes appeared on the monitor. A carotid pulse returned.

Almost as quickly as the bronchospasm had appeared and woke her from sleep, it disappeared. Within minutes she became easy to ventilate and she was taken to the ICU, sedated and on a ventilator. I told her parents the outlook was still extremely poor because of the length of time she had been without getting any oxygen and the likelihood was that she would have suffered a catastrophic brain injury which might lead to brain death.

This is what happened and the following day she became an organ donor. I hope her family gained some comfort from knowing that lives might have been saved or the quality of the lives of others might have been improved as a result of their daughter's generous gesture.

A colleague came in and we re-anaesthetised Jim and put him back on the ventilator. The following day he had a tracheostomy and within a week or so he was off the ventilator and later went home. Unfortunately, he started smoking again and over the next few years he steadily deteriorated to the extent that he was even breathless at rest. Walking from the living room to the kitchen would take several minutes, stopping every few yards to catch his breath. He was on frequent nebulisers and massive doses of steroids.

When he was again admitted to hospital one Friday afternoon four years after the ICU admission, apart from the severe dyspnoea – the sensation of breathlessness – he also had severe sciatica from a disc prolapse and was in excruciating pain from this. I was on call that day and suggested an epidural might help. I did this on the ward and within minutes he was pain-free. I again rang my wife's brothers and my wife's older sister in London to tell them that this time I felt he would die and if they wanted to see him they needed to come over as soon as possible. Her younger sister was somewhere in Paris on her first wedding anniversary and, in the days before mobile phones, she was uncontactable.

A colleague took over the on-call from Saturday morning and I explained to him and the consultant physician how Jim had been on a steady downward path for the last year in spite of being on all possible treatments for his COPD. To me, another period of ventilation was out of the question, there would be no point. It would only delay the inevitable: his death. I felt that the only course of action was for them to do their best to relieve his dyspnoea with diamorphine. I made it clear to the consultant physician and my anaesthetist colleague that the decision whether or not to ventilate him was theirs, not mine, but this was my own view of the situation. An infusion of diamorphine was started. An hour or two later I went to see him and he was smiling, a glass of whiskey in one hand and a lit cigarette in the other, drowsy from the effect of the opiate. Jim died peacefully the following night aged sixty-three, surrounded by his loving family.

Eighteen years later, history was repeating itself in a way. June, my mother-in-law had, like Jim, been on maximal medical treatment for many years for her asthma. Huge doses of steroids, inhalers, numerous courses of antibiotics, and like Jim she had a home nebuliser. In spite of this, her exercise tolerance had steadily deteriorated too. Shortly before she died, she stayed with us for a week or so. As with Jim, moving around the house would take time. Stopping every few yards to catch her breath and constantly in pain from severe osteoporosis caused by many years of massive steroid ingestion, it was clear to me that the end of her life was fast approaching.

She was admitted to a medical ward one Monday with pneumonia. I was in the theatre when I heard this, and when I finished the list I was told she might be transferred to the ICU. As with Jim, I knew that ventilating her would be pointless and would not alter the inevitable outcome. I, unlike all the other doctors in the hospital, had personally been able to see with my own eyes the inexorable worsening of her condition. I headed off to the ward hoping to talk to the consultant physician who was to be in charge of her care and also my anaesthetic colleague who had seen her earlier. I wanted them to know what I knew, although I was again aware that I couldn't interfere with any decisions about her care. I was too late. As I approached the ward I saw that June was in a bed being pushed by a porter and a nurse, on their way to the ICU. They had decided that non-invasive ventilation, or NIV, was indicated.

Before NIV became a treatment option for a patient with COPD, around fifteen years ago, the decision-making process was easier and more clear-cut. I'd often be asked to see this type of patient. They were almost always heavy smokers with frequent admissions to hospital with chest infections and on multiple medications including inhalers, steroids, sometimes home oxygen. They had very poor exercise tolerance and were often even breathless at rest or with minimal exertion. They often had symptoms of other diseases associated with smoking like ischaemic heart disease or cerebrovascular disease.

I'd be asked whether I felt the patient should be taken to the ICU and placed on a ventilator, when treatment on the ward had failed to improve their condition. It was often a difficult decision, and I'd often get an anaesthetic colleague to see the patient too if there was time. For some the decision was easier. If, for example, the patient was bed-bound, maybe having also had a stroke, in a nursing home, unhappy with their poor quality of life, on all the appropriate treatment for their chronic lung disease and still smoking heavily I would probably have felt that ventilation was not appropriate.

I've always been very wary of the term 'quality of life.' This is something only the patient themselves can really know. A doctor might feel a patient has a poor quality of life, but the patient might actually be quite happy with his or her life. They can quite understandably become angry when someone suggests they might have a poor quality of life. Although it might be hard for others to understand, some are happy with the hand they've been dealt.

There is a big difference between a patient who hasn't seen a doctor for years, smoking heavily and is on no drug treatment for COPD and one who is on every therapy imaginable and has been for a long period. There is a good chance with the former that if they are ventilated and subsequently seen by a respiratory physician, they stop smoking and are started on treatment they might be better than they have been for years. The other patient, though, has deteriorated in spite of all the treatment being given to try to prevent them reaching the stage of needing invasive ventilation. For them, there is less reserve and far less chance of success. As with much of medicine, however, things aren't all black and white.

I was on call one day and wandered into the ICU. One of my anaesthetic colleagues, who was very experienced but not a consultant, was drawing up drugs. A patient had just been admitted from ED with an acute exacerbation of COPD. She was so breathless she was unable to speak, with a very fast heart and respiratory rate and using accessory breathing muscles. These muscles in the neck are used subconsciously in an attempt to suck in more air. Normally the only muscles of respiration are the diaphragm, which lies between the chest and the abdomen, and the intercostals, in between the ribs. My colleague felt she was in respiratory failure and was about to put her on a ventilator. The nurse told me she'd been seen regularly in the chest clinic for many years. I examined her and suggested we wait a little longer and try another bronchodilator drug which hadn't yet been given, aminophylline. This drug has to be given slowly, over about fifteen minutes. I also gave her IV diamorphine for dyspnoea and explained that I thought things might still slowly improve. I then rang the chest physician to discuss her treatment prior to this admission. As soon as I gave him the patient's name he said whatever else I did, I shouldn't invasively ventilate her as she had end-stage disease, meaning she was expected to die soon. He felt she would never come off the breathing machine and be able to breathe for herself again. I was surprised as there had been several times when he and I had disagreed over whether a patient should be ventilated or not. He would often feel that they should be and I would feel the opposite as the outlook appeared to me to be hopeless. Now he was saying I shouldn't ventilate his patient. I told her what had been discussed but I also added I still thought she'd slowly improve and wouldn't need to go on a ventilator anyway. This is what happened and she slowly recovered. After a few days in the ICU she went to a ward. I saw her there every few days over the next few weeks before she was eventually discharged.

About four weeks later I was walking on the promenade in Douglas with my little grandson. A lady dressed in cycling gear and a helmet and goggles went flying past calling, 'Hi Keith, how's things?' I wondered if it could possibly be the same lady. About three weeks later I was in my local pub one evening. She came in with friends and insisted on buying me a drink to say thanks. She'd just returned from a three week holiday in Barbados, had started to exercise regularly, had stopped smoking and was feeling better than she had for years. When I later told the chest physician he was shocked as he'd all but written her off.

The decision I sometimes had to make was whether I take a patient to the ICU and put them on a ventilator or not. If not, I would ensure that diamorphine was available to relieve dyspnoea and a DNAR was completed so that if they should suffer a cardiac arrest no resuscitation would be started. I'd explain all of this to the patient and any close relatives, so everyone was aware.

If I felt ventilation in ICU was worth a try, in many cases I would put a limit on the time they would be on the ventilator. Resting the patient on a breathing machine, allowing the over-inflated lungs to deflate, allowing some time for antibiotics, steroids and other drugs to have an effect are all important. Remaining on a ventilator for weeks carries risks of muscle weakness and a deterioration in respiratory function.

I'd tell them that we'd try for maybe three days and then try to wake the patient and get them off the ventilator. In many cases this worked, and they made a good recovery. For those who were still unable to breathe on their own we would then usually aim to keep them as comfortable as possible with Diamorphine and allow them to die peacefully.

This sort of decision-making process changed with the development of NIV. Before this, all that was available was invasive ventilation, where the patient is anaesthetised and a tube inserted in the airway connected to the ventilator or keeping them comfortable and accepting they were probably going to die. With invasive ventilation, a patient is kept anaesthetised and the ventilator breathes for them. With NIV, instead of a tube, there is a tight-fitting face mask or nasal-mask, and this is attached by tubing to a ventilator which assists the patient's breathing. For many patients this is an excellent therapy.

Patients on NIV don't need to be anaesthetised, with all the potential problems associated with that. They can cough, eat and drink, communicate with doctors, nurses and relatives and NIV can often tide them over a period while their respiratory function improves. But there have been many times when I've said that I wished NIV had never been invented. These were on occasions when to me at least, it was being used inappropriately. Instead of being allowed to die peacefully and with dignity, some would spend days

If In Doubt

on NIV unnecessarily. One of the worst examples of the misuse of this therapy to me was unfortunately with June, my own mother-in-law.

A new term crept into common use about ten years ago: ceiling of care. This referred to the maximum level of invasive treatment appropriate for a particular patient. In June's case, my colleague who was responsible for admitting her to ICU and the consultant physician had decided invasive ventilation was not indicated as the chances of her surviving were negligible. However, a period of NIV was deemed to be of potential benefit. For the next two days she bravely tolerated the tight-fitting face mask and the high pressure forcing oxygen into her damaged lungs. Some patients can't tolerate it at all, it can become claustrophobic, painful and frightening. I am fairly certain I would be one of those patients. I probably wouldn't last more than a few minutes.

By the third day her oxygen requirements were going up and this correlated with a worsening of her chest X-ray appearance. Higher pressures were required to keep the oxygen in her blood at an adequate level. It was clear to me that she would not survive and about 3am the following morning a nurse in the ICU rang to say she wanted to talk to me. Driving in with my wife, I was fairly sure she was going to ask me what she thought she should do and I was preparing to tell her the truth – that as far as I was concerned, in spite of the NIV the situation was really bad, and I felt June had suffered enough and she needed to let go. I would promise her she'd be comfortable and peaceful at the end and she'd receive adequate amounts of diamorphine to ensure this happened.

When we arrived, the nurse said June had been asking for me, but when I went to her bedside, she didn't say the words I was expecting. She just chatted generally about how she was feeling, although with the noise from the ventilator, beeping alarms and the tight face mask it wasn't easy to hear what she was saying. We sat with her and my sister-in-law and her husband were also there. I told them I honestly felt she had been through enough and the outcome was inevitable. I was in an awkward position as a doctor. I couldn't interfere with any treatment she was receiving but I also couldn't simply say nothing if I felt she was receiving treatment I didn't agree with.

She continued to deteriorate and by Friday the X-ray was even worse, with even higher levels of oxygen being required. I asked a nurse to try to ensure she was kept as comfortable as possible with diamorphine. I had to leave the hospital for a couple of hours and at lunchtime I rang to enquire how she was doing. I was told a consultant physician had just seen her and felt she was too drowsy and this might be the diamorphine and he had crossed it off the prescription chart. I was furious and spoke to another anaesthetist and complained and he reinstated it immediately.

To me this was a situation that was out of control. She was suffering unnecessarily – I had no doubt about that. It was impossible for me to imagine she could survive and even if she did, the fact remained that just prior to her admission she was breathless on the most minimal exertion in spite of all the treatment she'd been taking for years. She was never going to be better than she had been before this admission, and I simply couldn't understand why none of my colleagues or the physician could see that and sit down with my wife and her sisters and explain that to them.

I spoke to the anaesthetist who was on call and said I felt I couldn't stand by and watch this any longer. He wasn't a consultant and although he agreed with me, he needed to discuss it with my consultant colleague who was on duty for ICU that day and the coming weekend. I asked him to speak to her daughters and explain the situation honestly and he did this. After they had spent some time with her, he took her off the ventilator, gave her the diamorphine and another drug to ensure she died peacefully and she died very quickly. At last, her suffering was over, and I was grateful to my colleague for that.

My own mother developed bowel cancer at the age of eighty-two. She had severe osteoporosis and Parkinson's disease and her mobility had become poor, with generalised arthritic pain. She had once told me she 'didn't think much of this growing old lark' and often wished she could go off to sleep and not wake up.

My sister, Lynn, a medical secretary in Durham, rang to say mam was being lined up for surgery in her hospital. They were planning an operation to remove part of the large bowel. Lynn knew the consultant surgeon and had asked him if he would talk to me about the operation. He rang me and I told him my own view of the situation. Mam was very weak by then and I told him she had had enough of life. He said he was pleased we had spoken as he was wondering himself if he was doing the right thing in operating. She didn't have the op. She rapidly deteriorated and was admitted to a ward where a diamorphine infusion was started. By the time I travelled back to the hospital in Durham from the island she was unconscious. She died peacefully a few days later.

A few years after that, my dad developed bowel cancer. He was then eighty-nine and I also had serious reservations about him having surgery and told Lynn this. I arrived back in the same hospital where my sister worked, and my mother had died, a few hours before he was due to go for his operation. I met the surgeon and she felt surgery was a reasonable option, so I said nothing.

We later saw him in the ICU after the operation and after a day there he returned to the ward. For the first couple of weeks he did well, then suddenly became ill with pain and vomiting. By then I was back on the island and Lynn rang while I was in theatre one day to tell me that a scan had revealed he had a leaking aortic aneurysm. The aneurysm – a weakness in the main artery as it passed down the back of the abdominal cavity close to the spine –was known about but now the leak meant it would rupture and patients with this usually died from massive blood loss.

A few years earlier there would have been no question of surgery for someone of my dad's age and general state of health. But a relatively new procedure was then being performed. Instead of major abdominal surgery an Endovascular Aneurysm Repair (EVAR) could be carried out in many cases. This involved inserting a graft to bypass the leak through a small incision in the groin, using X-rays to correctly position it. Lynn told me a surgeon had seen him and he was being prepared for the procedure. I told her I thought he shouldn't have it. As with my mother I felt he had been through enough and should be allowed to die peacefully. The surgeon rang about an hour later and I explained this. He, like the surgeon who was to do my mother's surgery, was also unsure about whether to go ahead but he felt it was reasonable to do so. He had spoken at length with my dad and said he had seemed to understand the options available to him. Still in my own operating theatre on the island, my sister rang shortly after that to say he had gone to theatre.

Again, as with his first operation he initially seemed to be doing ok but then there was a rapid deterioration, with increasing frailty. About six weeks later my youngest daughter and I arrived at his house near Durham one Friday evening. He was in bed, and he'd had nothing to eat for three days and was refusing any liquids apart from sips of water. She told him he needed to eat to keep up his strength and asked why he was refusing food. I knew what his answer would be.

'Because I want to die.'

He was trying to speed up his own death. Two nights later his condition had worsened, and I knew he would die that night. I fell asleep on the settee next to him – his bed had been moved downstairs as he was too weak to climb the stairs. Around 3am he was asleep and appeared to be breathing comfortably and I went up to bed. At about 5am I woke up and walked halfway down the stairs and listened. I could hear him breathing. I went back up to bed and fell asleep again. At 8am I went back down. He was dead.

Many years earlier I'd told my medical school friends about him. He was my best friend and I'd always tried to be like him. I was sad he'd died but happy that he had died at home and he'd at last found peace.

CHAPTER 13

Death

I must have seen thousands of dead bodies during my career – on my first day at medical school I saw about forty in the dissection room. It was almost as if that ancient tradition, on the first day, was there to begin the process of making us almost become inured to death as soon as possible.

As if there was no time to lose, we needed to face it quickly. Maybe they were even trying to weed out a few of us already on day one? After all, death was going to be a big part of our lives from now on if we wanted to be doctors. What better way than this? Forty corpses in one room with one hundred and fifty brand new medical students.

My first experience involving death – after my earliest memory of believing my mother had died – was when I was about eight. My dad had taken my brother and I one evening to see his mother. When we got there the door was open but she was out. We waited maybe an hour, watching TV, wondering where she was. When she came back she told my dad she'd been to a neighbour's house to 'lay someone out'. For a few seconds I had a vision of her, our lovely grandmother aged about sixty, angrily storming round and punching a neighbour, knocking them out cold. My brother and I looked at each other. She explained that whenever someone who lived nearby died, a relative would ask her to lay out the body, preparing it for the undertaker. My dad later told us she'd been doing this for many years. Whenever someone died at home in the streets close to her own, they'd call on my grandmother and she'd always go to help. When I was seventeen, I saw her own body laid out in her bedroom, just before her funeral, the first dead body I'd ever seen.

If In Doubt

A few years later when I worked as a nursing auxiliary during my year before going off to medical school there were a few dead bodies on the elderly patient wards, or villas as they were known. There were some during our training as we'd follow the house officer around when on call. He'd be called to certify death so the body could be moved to the mortuary.

In the final year of training, we were allowed a week off from studies, if we wished, to work as a locum house officer. We'd be paid to step in when a house officer was on leave. It was a way to gain experience and help prepare us for the day we ourselves would start work after qualifying from medical school. I decided I'd like to do this, although I was terrified really, and spent a week in St Catherine's Hospital in Birkenhead as a medical house officer.

On the first day there were several admissions and my job was to clerk them. This involved taking a history, asking about their illness, getting an idea of their background, examining them and coming up with a differential diagnosis, or some possible conditions that might be present.

I'd order relevant investigations, take blood samples, order X-rays. I'd inform the senior house officer next up in rank to me about my proposed plan and he would review the patient himself. During that morning I was examining a patient when a nurse asked if I'd see the man in the next bed. He'd just been admitted from A&E complaining of chest pain and sudden shortness of breath.

I told her I'd be there shortly. A few minutes later she was back.

'I think you should come now,' she said, holding the curtain open for me, staring. Waiting, eyebrows raised.

'Please?'

The man, about sixty, tall and slim, grey-haired, was sitting up in bed, an oxygen mask covering most of his face. Dried vomit smeared his grey jumper, the smell almost making me retch. He was breathing very fast, secretions rattling in his throat, too weak to clear them.

I'd hear that 'death rattle' again many, many times.

Starting to go through the questions I'd carefully rehearsed, he didn't speak. He couldn't, too exhausted from the sheer effort of breathing. Within a minute or so his breathing started to slow as his eyes slowly closed. He became unresponsive and I put my hand on his shoulder, gently shaking him. Nothing. This was definitely not supposed to happen. I felt, and was, completely useless, not knowing what to say or do. Fortunately, at that moment the nurse was back.

'Shall I call the team?

'Please,' I replied, trying to appear calm. As if I knew what was happening, like I'd been in this situation many times. No need to panic, it was all under control. I don't think she was fooled. What now?

All medical students today become proficient in CPR, or cardio-pulmonary resuscitation. They practice on mannequins in simulators, perfecting their skills. Most pass the Advanced Life Support Course, while they are still students. We'd had a tutorial or two but had seen very few cardiac arrests during our medicine attachments. As I was trying to decide what to do, the bed space seemed to fill with doctors and nurses and I felt as if I was being slowly forced backwards. Which is in fact what was happening. I stood and watched, saying nothing.

CPR started.

'What's the story?' the SHO asked, as he attached red, green and yellow leads to the man's chest.

'I don't know, he's just arrived from A&E complaining of chest pain. I was just starting to see him when he arrested.'

The anaesthetist inserted a cannula into a vein in his neck in seconds and an ECG was attached so they could identify the heart rhythm and a defibrillator was brought to the bedside and switched on, ready. Cardiac arrests are classed as shockable if a defibrillator is indicated or non-shockable if it is not. The shockable ones have by far the best chance of a good outcome. Within seconds the heart can often be re-started. The patient can literally come back to life and make a complete recovery in a split second. A defibrillator passes an electrical current across the heart which stops all electrical activity. In many cases the heart miraculously starts itself back up again, but only if the ECG shows VF (ventricular fibrillation) or VT (ventricular tachycardia).

Defibrillation, or shocking, is useless in asystole or PEA (pulseless electrical activity), the other two patterns seen during a cardiac arrest. This fact is the main reason for the existence of coronary care units. Continuously monitored with an ECG, if a patient suddenly develops a shockable rhythm they can be defibrillated immediately.

'Stop for a second!'

A wavy line on the monitor screen. No complexes, the regular spikes seen with a normal trace. Asystole, the worst type of cardiac arrest with a very poor outlook, no need for the defibrillator yet.

The anaesthetist injected intravenous adrenaline through the line in his neck. I watched the resuscitation for twenty minutes or so. There was no sense of panic, no raised voices, everyone was calm and I was in awe of the anaesthetist and SHO. Will I ever be able to do that, I wondered. Take control, be calm, make the right decisions, save lives? At that moment I doubted it. After twenty minutes they felt it was hopeless and resuscitation stopped. I had done precisely nothing. In fact, I had done worse than nothing. When the nurse had first asked me to see him, she'd been worried but I'd waited a few minutes until she'd come to ask again. If I'd gone immediately maybe I'd have called for help earlier? Maybe he wouldn't have died?

I felt bad that I'd messed up already, hours into the locum. In the office I made a note of what had happened and certified his death. The doctors left.

'Are you going to tell his family?' a nurse asked.

'Oh shit,' I thought, 'I've never done this before.'

I prepared myself and rehearsed what I'd say. His son had just arrived on the ward. He was in the visitors' room and stood up as I walked in and offered his hand. He was in tears. Tall, his glistening thick black hair slicked back, white overalls covered in every colour of paint imaginable. His trainers were multi-coloured too. The call telling him about his dad had sent him rushing straight to hospital from his work. I introduced myself and explained that his father had probably had a heart attack and suffered a cardiac arrest and sadly had died. I was sorry. He said he appreciated all we'd done and felt bad for me as I'd had to tell him the bad news. I felt ashamed.

'He's thanking me,' I thought after I'd delayed seeing his dad, and then when his heart stopped I'd still done nothing at all. I averted my eyes from the nurse, the same one who'd asked for my help and didn't get it. Did she blame me?

That night I'd arranged to meet a friend of our family from Stanley. His father and mine were best friends for many years and he was working in Birkenhead. We were in a pub when a familiar face appeared. The son of the man who had died earlier had walked into the pub. He spotted me immediately and walked over.

'I want to buy you a drink, and say thanks again for everything.'

I felt embarrassed. I could hardly tell him the truth.

'I want to thank you for all you did for my dad, thanks for trying your best.'

He insisted he buy us both a pint and I thanked him and wished him well.

A few months later, now a house officer, I'd often be called to confirm death, often in the middle of the night. In the now quiet, darkened ward, a dead body would be surrounded by the bodies of sleeping, snoring patients.

If a cardiac arrest call had been made, they'd have been rudely awakened by the commotion. Moving shadows on the wall and ceiling cast by the illuminated bedspace. The curtains constantly moving as nurses and doctors brush past, silhouetted for the anxious onlookers. I think most, unless they were completely deaf, would realise what was happening. Out of respect, I suppose, I have never once heard anyone complain about noise and their disturbed sleep. In that situation I've always tried to be as quiet as possible. Others often don't give it a second thought. At times the din is almost deafening, several people talking at once, louder and louder to be heard above the others. Beeping from the ECG machine. Opening and closing of drawers in the metal trolley, the cracking open of glass ampoules, tearing open sterile packages. The bed creaking under the strain of the chest compressions.

Even with the din surrounding them, the chest compressor, perhaps silently singing along to *Stayin' Alive* by the Bee Gees, keeping up a steady hundred compressions per minute, in time with the beat.

'Coming up to two minutes, get ready to check rhythm and pulse.'

'Two minutes.'

Chest compressions stop for the absolute minimum time, hands stay where they are on the chest, ready, waiting. Every second counts. All eyes turn to the screen on the monitor.

'There's no pulse.'

'Still asystole, resume chest compressions.'

And so it goes on until either the heart restarts or it becomes futile to continue. If anyone disagrees they try for another few two-minute cycles but everyone will know by then the chances of a successful outcome are miniscule.

Even if the heart re-starts the chances of an anoxic brain injury are very high as a brain deprived of oxygen even for four or five minutes is at risk of irreversible damage.

Automatic defibrillators give instructions to let the person in charge of it know whether it should be used. More noise for the silent audience, like a voice from a Dr Who Dalek.

'Analysing rhythm, stand clear, analysing rhythm, stand clear.'

Silence for a few seconds, then:

'Shock advised, deliver shock, shock advised, deliver shock.'

The whirring, high pitched sound as it charges. A miniature air raid siren.

A thud as the body jolts in the bed.

Before the body can be moved someone, usually the house officer, would need to confirm death. Look for any signs of life. Listen with a stethoscope for heart sounds, caused by the closing of the valves, usually described in our medical books as 'lub-dup, lub-dup, lub dup.' Use a bright torch light to see if the dilated pupils react. Normally the pupil constricts to reduce the amount of light passing through it. Death means they will be apnoeic, not breathing, with absent heart sounds and have fixed pupils which don't react to light.

There would be a discussion about the cause of death if known. If any doubt remained as to the cause, or it was a sudden and unexpected death the coroner would need to be informed. The coroner would decide if a post-mortem was required or even an inquest to determine what had caused the person to die.

There are never any cardiac arrest calls in the hospice.

For the first eighteen years or so of my consultant post I'd occasionally be asked to see patients there. When the switchboard operator would ring me to say the hospice was after me, I felt happy. This, to me, was one of the most rewarding parts of the job.

The hospice doctors would have followed their palliative pain pathway, starting with simple analgesics with few unpleasant side effects: paracetamol, non-steroidals such as ibuprofen. Then gradually adding in other drugs known to help with certain types of pain. Until we appointed an anaesthetist with an interest in chronic pain, about fifteen years into my consultant post, I'd often be asked to help.

If pain was confined to one part of the body a regional nerve block might be indicated. Local anaesthetic is given by a steady infusion from a syringe pump and delivered to nerves supplying that part of the body. I'd take advice from pain specialists at Walton in Liverpool or in Clatterbridge on the Wirral. The patients would be usually suffering from metastatic cancer, cancer that has spread, perhaps to bone or the spine, compressing and infiltrating nerves. An epidural or other nerve block could in some cases take away the pain completely, allowing a reduction in the dose of opiate drugs with all of their unpleasant side effects. Although no treatment might be possible for the underlying condition the quality of life for the patient might be dramatically improved.

Deaths in the hospice were anticipated, expected. A DNAR would be discussed with every patient so that all were clear that no resuscitation would take place. The sole aim of the doctors, nurses and psychologists and others involved with end-of-life care is to try to give the patient the best possible death they could have. Balancing the side effects of drugs against their effectiveness in relieving pain or relief of dyspnoea, the feeling of being breathless, is tricky.

I've always felt that making any sort of prediction about when death might occur is fraught with danger for a doctor. Having made several hopelessly inaccurate guesses earlier in my career I'd become very wary when asked,

'How long has he got, Doctor?'

I long ago learnt that lesson. From then on, if I was asked the question I'd choose my words very carefully.

Often I'd hear that a patient had been told they had a finite time, say six weeks. I've never understood why this still happens. No matter how experienced a doctor might be, the fact remains that it is impossible to say when a person will die in many situations. The exception to this though is when that doctor is an experienced oncologist, a cancer specialist. I can still recall several patients now in the hospice. All had metastatic cancer. I'd been asked to advise whether I could improve their pain management with some kind of regional, local anaesthetic block.

The patient, having often been practically unconscious from the effects of the sedative and opiate analgesics like diamorphine, would seemingly miraculously come back to life. After my block the drugs would be reduced or stopped. They weren't needed, for now.

Pain-free, without the need for these sedating drugs, they'd be chatting away with their families, smiling, eating delicious food prepared by the hospice chef. I always thought they looked as good as any meal I'd seen in a top restaurant. There'd be a brief feeling of guilt, feeling slightly jealous of them, thinking of what awaited later me in the hospital canteen.

It was all an illusion though.

The cancer was still there, death still inevitable and imminent. The complete turnaround in the appearance of the patient, though, could fool the unwary. True, the quality of life might be better now. The quality of death remained to be seen.

The nurse would always greet me with a cheery smile. Had it tricked her too?

'Hi Keith, he's doing great now! Off for a home visit soon to see his grandkids, he's so much better, still pain-free. Your epidural's been brilliant! You can come again!'

If the drugs he'd been on earlier had continued he might have died peacefully a week or two earlier and a relative might now feel some kind of miraculous recovery was in the making.

The visiting oncologist however would remind everyone of the reality.

Their own hospital, Clatterbridge, was on the Wirral. From Liverpool, once a week, it was literally a flying visit.

Their day would be spent seeing new and follow up patients in the clinic in the hospital before heading back to the airport. With barely time for a coffee, they'd still try to spare a few minutes to nip across to the hospice, a three-minute walk away. Their itinerary in the hospice would have been pre-planned for them so no time would be wasted.

It was difficult to believe, even for me, that a patient who now looked so good would die so quickly, but the oncologist was usually correct with their own prediction.

Or at least very close.

I became involved in Simon's care when he was admitted to the ED with a very high temperature and low blood pressure, rapid heart rate. He was sixteen, about to start A-levels, the same age as one of my daughters. Suffering from a rare form of leukaemia made him susceptible to infection. A fairly mild chest infection had now spread into his blood, causing septicaemic shock. Resuscitation with IV fluids had been commenced. IV antibiotics would be the main treatment, after blood had been taken for culture which would hopefully identify the bacteria. If the antibiotic is given before the blood is taken it may prove impossible to ever identify the cause. In spite of this, after three hours his blood pressure was so low a risk of organ failure became a concern and I decided he needed treatment in the ICU. IV drugs to support his circulation were needed to prevent his kidneys from failing. He made a good recovery, and that incident was the start of a long relationship for him and his family.

For me becoming personally involved with some patients has been very rewarding, as I'm sure most doctors have found. With any patient, be it an eighty-year-old with a hip fracture needing an anaesthetic or a toddler with pneumonia, my basic approach has always been the same. I think, subconsciously, the vast majority of doctors do the same. I'd tried to put myself in the position of the son or daughter of the elderly patient or the parents of the toddler.

If In Doubt

'What would I want if I were them?'

If I can answer my own question by providing what I would want myself, that is probably as much as I can do; the best I can offer.

For a patient with a condition that might go on for months or years I might feel that I'd also like someone who I could turn to for advice at any time, who is straight and honest and genuinely cares and wants to help.

Simon became one such patient. I received calls from his mother via the hospital while on holiday in Tenerife, in a black cab in London as we rode past the Tower of London on our way to our hotel and on weekends when I wasn't on call. She'd ask for advice and needed help and I hope I gave her that every time.

At the end, two years after we'd first met, I'd visit him each day in the hospice. The nurses had managed to find a room for him with an adjoining one for his brother and sister. They were similar in age to him; he was now eighteen. His condition had steadily deteriorated to the extent they'd all felt hospice care would be best for him. They felt that might be better for him than caring for him at home, although this had been a difficult decision.

He began his end-of-life care pathway.

Sedative drugs and painkillers were given, titrated to try to get right for that balance between comfort and unpleasant side effects. When he stopped eating and drinking his family would try to keep his mouth moist with swabs dipped in water and small sips. They'd decided they were staying with him and slept in the hospice each night.

I was due to go on leave for a week to our apartment in Tenerife so I said my goodbyes and told his mum I'd keep in touch with the nurses while away. I rang two or three times and asked the nurses to tell his family I was thinking of them. When I got back I rang again. He was still there, although slowly deteriorating, deeply unconscious. He'd had nothing to eat or drink for around nine days, and as was the policy in the hospice, he was receiving no intravenous fluids. When I went to see him later that day he didn't look a lot different than when I'd last seen him. His family were still with him.

'This is so wrong, Keith.' His mum had tears in her eyes. 'I realise you can't do anything but this can't be right, can it? You wouldn't treat an animal like this.'

I felt at a loss to know what to say to her, but I agreed that surely there had to be a better way of allowing someone a peaceful death than this?

I again called in every night after work, not really knowing what to say to them. In these situations there was always a dilemma. Should I stop going altogether? If I did that would they think I'd deserted them at the end and think badly of me? When I did go, though, I never really knew what to say. Might they feel I was intruding into their grief? I knew this wasn't really an issue but the thought wouldn't go away. I felt that as a doctor I was failing Simon and his family in some way. How could we allow this to go on, I wondered, knowing that in his case it was a certainty he would die soon and his family were going through the agony of watching this seemingly never-ending suffering? Another seven days passed before he died.

Euthanasia means 'easy death.' In a book such as this there is not the space to discuss the ins and outs, rights and wrongs. My own views are irrelevant, but I have often wondered if in the future there will be major changes to the way we care for many patients who are at the end of their lives. A recent article in The Guardian, in 2019, reported:

The British Social Attitudes survey, published in 2017, sheds light on views about voluntary euthanasia, showing that people generally support the idea of doctors ending the life of a terminally ill person who requests it (78%), but that there is less support for a close relative doing the job (39%). It also shows that fervent support for voluntary euthanasia was lower if the person in question has a non-terminal illness or is dependent on relatives for all their needs but not terminal or in pain.

If In Doubt

I hope that at some point in the future there will be a way to have a peaceful and dignified way of dying for some of those for whom life has become intolerable and there is no prospect of it improving.

A stroke, or cerebrovascular accident (CVA), occurs when the blood supply to a part of the brain is interrupted. The brain cells rapidly die within minutes if they receive no oxygen and nutrients, so, as with a heart attack, or myocardial infarction, urgent treatment is required.

Malignant MCA (middle cerebral artery) syndrome was a term I'd never even heard of when I was asked one evening when I was on call to see a forty-seven-year-old lady, Debbie.

A secretary in a law firm, she'd been treated for high blood pressure for several years and was a smoker. Both of these increase the chances of stroke. Three days earlier she'd woken to discover a right-sided weakness of her arm and leg. A brain scan confirmed a large stroke. During the previous day she'd complained of worsening headaches and nausea, vomiting several times and being unable to keep any food down. A second CT scan showed a massive area of infarction – dead brain tissue with oedema surrounding it and midline shift.

The skull is like an enclosed box. The only way into it, apart from small holes (foramina) for blood vessels, is a hole at the base, the foramen magnum. The upper continuation of the spinal cord, the medulla oblongata, passes through it, the junction of spinal cord and brain. If the pressure within the skull rises from brain swelling, bleeding into or around it for example, the pressure can cause compression of the medulla and the nerves and blood vessels passing through the foramen magnum. In some cases, the whole brain can die, or infarct. This condition is termed brain death.

The swelling on one side of the brain, if severe, can push the midline of the brain across to the other side and this pressure causes a decrease in blood supply to that normal brain tissue.

In Malignant MCA Syndrome, swelling around the infarcted brain can cause a rapid neurological deterioration. 80% of patients die from the condition. In some early cases surgery can be attempted, a decompressive hemicraniectomy, where part of the skull is removed to 'open the closed box' and allow the brain to expand out and reduce the dangerous rise in pressure that would otherwise occur. The bone flap is stored under sterile conditions and returned to its original position later if the patient survives. One of the risks of surgery is that the patient might survive but have a severe neurological deficit. With Debbie, surgery wasn't an option. Her CT scan had been seen by neurosurgeons at Walton, the regional centre for neurosurgery. They advised she should have conservative treatment.

By now her conscious level had fallen and her eyes were permanently closed. There was no movement in her right arm and leg and she gave no indication that she could hear when spoken to. The consultant physician had spoken to a neurologist at Walton who felt the outcome was extremely poor. The concern now was that she was unlikely to be able to protect her airway. It might become obstructed and also she might vomit and some of that might pass into her lungs. The question I was asked was:

'What should we do? Should she be intubated and ventilated?'

As with surgery, ventilating her to ensure her lungs remained uncontaminated and she was receiving enough oxygen with a clear airway meant again she might survive but with a severe neurological deficit. She might never wake up, remaining in a persistent vegetative state which to most, certainly to me, would be even worse than death.

After seeing her and a long discussion with the consultant physician I said I'd keep calling back to review her during the night and think about the best way forward. I went back every hour or so – I'd told the nurses I'd be in my office, playing my guitar as usual, if they needed me and left my phone number. It was going to be another long night. I wanted to see whether the general trend was one of gradual improvement or deterioration. I also spoke to the hospital's stroke specialist to see if he had any experience with this condition. He felt that with the massive area of infarcted brain on the scan, the chances of her surviving were very small.

Even if she didn't die or become brain dead, he felt there would almost certainly be a very severe neurological deficit as a result of the other side of the brain being damaged too. It was time for another talk with her family, her husband and twin sons, who were about twenty. Together we went over the options available to us and the consultant physician and I both felt that if we anaesthetised her and put her on a ventilator we'd lose the ability to assess her neurologically, most importantly her conscious level. We both felt the risk of her never waking up once we tried to take off the ventilator after stopping the sedation was very high. So did the neurologist at Walton. That might mean weeks, months, even years of misery for the family. I felt that if she deteriorated further the outcome would then be so poor she should not be put on a ventilator. I completed a DNAR.

In these very difficult situations, I've always liked a few hours to think about the various options. Taking advice from my anaesthetic colleagues is useful too. I've often rang other anaesthetists in Liverpool too for advice – some have been friends from medical school. For an important one like this I always felt I needed all the help I could get, although it would be my decision and I would need to justify it if a complaint was later made. At the end of the day though, or in this case, at the start of the day – it was now 7am – I had to make a decision.

I felt we should take her to the ICU so she could be watched continuously. I'd insert a nasogastric tube, a tube through her nose into her stomach and have it aspirated hourly to reduce the risk of her aspirating gastric contents – having liquid from her stomach passing into her lungs. I was also concerned that her airway was at risk. There had been a few episodes overnight of obstruction as she was unable to keep it open as someone who is fully conscious would do automatically. I inserted a nasopharyngeal airway, a soft plastic tube passed into the nostril which is usually effective in keeping the upper airway patent.

Apart from oxygen and some IV fluids, that was as far as I felt we should go. I'd watched her closely overnight and had come to the conclusion that she was slowly deteriorating. I didn't feel invasive ventilation, anaesthetising her and putting a tube into her trachea then putting her on a ventilator was indicated. Her family, I hoped, could see I'd given it a lot of thought and taken advice from others. I've always felt this to be important.

Although they were clearly very upset and worried, they seemed to accept our plan. One of her sons was crying uncontrollably and he left the room, apologising as he walked past me.

Some consultants seem to think it is some kind of sign of failure or weakness to have to ask advice before making a decision. For an important one like this I always felt I needed all the help I could get, although it would be my decision and I would need to justify it if a complaint was later made. In the ICU I handed over her care to my colleagues; much of their work was in intensive care medicine. Fortunately, they felt my decision was reasonable. Over the next three days there was a slight improvement and it was felt that she could again be cared for back on the ward. I spoke to her family again and saw her over the next few days before I had a week of annual leave.

About three weeks after my break, I'd just finished anaesthetising for an emergency caesarean section one evening around 9pm. As I left the obstetric unit to walk back to my office I walked past ward seven, where Debbie had been a patient. I stopped. Should I go in and enquire what eventually happened to her? Then I went to the desk where three nurses sat chatting. I told them I'd helped look after her and was wondering if they could tell me what happened, dreading the worst, thinking she'd probably died. They looked at each other, not saying anything for a few seconds. One turned to me:

'Come and see for yourself.'

She took me to a four-bedded bay in which there was only one patient. Sat on the edge of the bed, in red and white striped pyjamas and reading a book, was a lady I didn't recognise. I looked at the nurse, who smiled and walked back to her colleagues. I checked the chart at the end of the bed. It was Debbie.

I explained who I was and a little of what had happened. She couldn't remember anything of coming into hospital or anything of her first week or so after her admission. Her speech was normal. She proudly showed me her hands, making fists, raising her arms above her head, the exercises the physiotherapist had shown her. Touching the tips of her fingers with the tip of the thumb on the same hand.

'It's getting better every day now. The right arm was very weak when I woke up, but I'm getting there,' she said smiling. There was no asymmetry of her face, no weakness there.

'Can you walk okay?' I asked.

She stood up and walked across the bay and back.

I was amazed and I told her that. Whether my decisions were right or wrong, she'd made a remarkable recovery.

'I'm going home tomorrow,' she said.

CHAPTER 14

Changes

I've seen many changes in the way anaesthetists work during my thirty-seven-year career, some good and some not so good. Drugs, anaesthetic equipment, therapies used in intensive care, training, the way major trauma is managed now –the list goes on and on.

For some anaesthetists, their work involves only cardiac anaesthesia or perhaps paediatric or neuro-anaesthesia. Some only work as chronic pain doctors, seeing patients in clinics and sometimes in the hospice setting. Others might work only in intensive care medicine, or the majority of their time might be spent in an obstetric unit.

As there is only one general hospital on the Isle of Man for a population of around 85,000 my own duties involved many different subspecialties. That was one of the reasons I wanted to work there in the first place –the variety of work appealed to me although in many ways it meant that the job was harder and more stressful. My colleagues and I needed to be prepared for almost anything at any time.

There might be a patient with major trauma or a toddler with severe meningitis. An emergency caesarean section in the middle of the night or difficult ethical decisions in the ICU, transferring a seriously ill patient to Liverpool on a small plane. We might be asked to help with the resuscitation of a new-born baby. Literally anything could happen.

This meant that instead of having to keep up to date with only one or two of the various branches of the specialty, like major trauma, obstetrics or intensive care, we had to do our best to keep up with them all. I often thought it was like trying to keep plates spinning on poles at the same time, something I remember seeing on an episode of Blue Peter when I was about ten. He was rushing from one to another, tweaking them to stop plates falling and shattering, trying to get his name into the Guinness Book of World records.

In order to help me stay abreast of managing sick young children or patients suffering trauma I became an instructor on the Advanced Paediatric Life Support course (APLS) and the Advanced Trauma Life Support (ATLS) courses. I did this for the final fifteen years or so of my career. Apart from the satisfaction of teaching and passing on some of my experiences to young doctors, it increased my confidence in looking after patients with conditions I might only encounter rarely.

An example of a major change during my career is in the management of major trauma. As a junior doctor there was no real system for dealing with this kind of patient. Since the early 1980s the ATLS course, and more recently other similar courses, have taught doctors the ABCDE approach. It teaches a safe and reliable method for immediate management of trauma patients. The same basic concept also applies to the APLS and ALS (Advanced Life Support) courses. The basic principles are assessing the patient rapidly in a structured way and dealing with life-threatening injuries first, as they are detected, in order to save life.

Critically ill patients coming into hospital are often brought in by a paramedic. In March 2020 I contacted the local newspapers to explain that I was retiring soon after thirty years as a consultant. For many years I'd wanted to try to raise awareness of the fantastic work the paramedics do but I was running out of time and I asked if they would consider an article explaining this. It was published as a double page spread and in it I wrote my own 'personal tribute' to the paramedics.

If In Doubt

For many years I'd been a member of the Paramedic Steering Committee and was often, along with my anaesthetic colleagues, involved in teaching them airway skills and IV cannulation in the operating theatre. They would also have mannikins to practice these life-saving interventions on but here was a chance to have a 'hands-on' session. Tracheal intubation, insertion of LMAs and IGELS and airway-opening manoeuvres on real patients could be carried out after the patients had been anaesthetised, with their consent.

Many of the patients they'd transported to hospital would require a period of intensive care, and I've always thought it slightly unfair that it is often the ICU staff and anaesthetists and surgeons who might get credit for looking after the patient but the paramedic's contribution, because it happened so early on in the chain of events, is often easily forgotten. Examples of these types of patients with potentially life-threatening conditions are out-of-hospital cardiac arrests, trauma - such as head, chest or pelvic injury, severe epileptic seizures and patients who are suffering from drug overdoses.

A Paramedic Science/Practice Degree is required to qualify. Paramedics normally work in a team of two, with one paramedic supported by an ambulance technician, emergency medical technician or emergency care assistant. On some occasions, though, they work alone from an emergency response car. They have a very difficult and stressful job, at times having to make life-and-death decisions in seconds. As well as having to deal with the patient they also need to interact with their relatives or friends, who may be aggressive or highly emotional. I recall several tragic incidents, one of them around midnight while I was working in Newcastle about thirty years ago. After handing over the care of a patient who'd been a pillion passenger on a motorbike and had sustained a serious head injury and obvious bilateral femur fractures, the paramedic took me aside so no-one else could hear.

'It was horrific', he explained. 'The motorcyclist was probably doing well over a hundred miles an hour. He'd lost control on a bend and smashed head-on into a motorhome. He was decapitated and his arm was wedged behind the bumper of the van, amputated. We had to evacuate the couple and their five-year-old daughter from the motorhome as soon as possible, as there was smoke coming from the engine compartment and the bike was basically a fireball a few yards away. I tried to shield the child from the sight but I'm not sure if I managed'? Then he was off to another job, details of which suddenly came through on his radio as we spoke.

I have worked with many people in other roles in the hospital who I know would be so traumatised - or say they were - if they'd been involved in this sort of incident. They would possibly go off for months with 'stress'. For the paramedic, always professional, there was no question of that happening. He took it all in his stride, clearly upset but accepting it as part of his job. He didn't expect or want any sympathy; there were no tears of self-pity.

Anaesthetists work in warm, well-lit surroundings, with colleagues close by if needed; ODP's and other anaesthetists; surrounded by medical equipment. Paramedics simply don't have these luxuries and I was always impressed with their calmness and professionalism when handing over the care of a patient in A&E. Much of our job as anaesthetists had usually already been done by them - the airway would be secured often with a tracheal tube and if there was a risk of a cervical spine injury, a collar would also have been fitted to stabilise the neck and hopefully lessen the risk of further possible damage during transfer. There would be a hand-written account of the incident, their initial findings and the likely mechanism of injury -which can give clues to the likely trauma sustained. Any drugs they'd given, or IV fluid, details of the tracheal tube and IV cannula would be documented.

If In Doubt

For anyone considering a job that is interesting although stressful but of vital importance and very rewarding with a 'hands-on' approach in literally saving lives then to me they need look no further than a potential career as a paramedic. They have always been unsung heroes as far as I am concerned - I hope I have got across the respect I feel for them all.

In any trauma patient the first priority is to ensure there is a patent airway, A. An unconscious patient can die in minutes if the airway is obstructed. It may only require a simple manoeuvre like a jaw thrust to achieve this airway opening. Next, breathing, B, is assessed. If a patient isn't breathing adequately this has to be assisted, preferably with 100% oxygen rather than air which only contains 21%. C stands for circulation. If a patient is bleeding, firm pressure might help to stem the flow but urgent surgery might be required. Replacement of the lost blood will require intravenous lines and cross matching of blood. D means disability and refers to the conscious level, of particular importance in a head injury. Exposure, E, refers to the part of the assessment where all clothing is removed while at the same time trying to keep the patient warm to look for injuries.

There are major trauma centres now. For the Isle of Man this means such patients are swiftly transferred by plane to Aintree or the Royal in Liverpool. There have been many changes in the management of major trauma over the last ten years or so. For a patient with massive blood loss, say from a fractured pelvis or from blood loss into the chest multiple rib fractures the initial management would usually include large volumes of crystalloid IV fluids. This is basically water with dissolved salts in it. As an initial way of restoring the volume of lost blood this was felt to be an appropriate treatment until blood could be cross-matched and given.

In recent years this approach has been shown to be detrimental.

During a period of blood loss, the body's natural response is to vasoconstrict or narrow small blood vessels. This has the effect of squeezing down on the blood remaining in the blood vessels and is a way of maintaining oxygen-carrying blood to vital organs, in particular the brain. Clots form on the damaged blood vessel wall in an attempt to plug the hole and reduce or completely halt any blood loss. Clotting factors are required and red cells are used up during this process. While all of this is going on, fluid starts to pass from around the cells surrounding the vessels into the blood itself in an attempt to restore the circulating volume.

If a large volume of clear fluid is given intravenously, the remaining clotting factors are diluted, meaning blood doesn't form clots as efficiently. In a massive haemorrhage the blood pressure may be low. If this suddenly increases as IV fluids are given rapidly the clots may become dislodged and bleeding may re-start. The term 'pop the clot' has sometimes been used to describe this phenomenon, the blood clot being forced off the damaged blood vessel wall by the sudden rise in pressure. This leads to further haemorrhage. If the IV fluid is cold, this also increases the risk of reduced blood clotting, known as coagulopathy. Because of this warm IV fluids are kept in EDs or warming devices are used to rapidly heat infused fluids.

The current management of these seriously injured patients is to give minimal, if any, IV fluids apart from blood. Now the emphasis is on rapidly establishing where the blood is being lost and stopping it as soon as possible, usually through urgent surgery. Whereas a few years ago years ago the patient would be rapidly resuscitated to get the low blood pressure back towards a normal level, it is now generally felt that accepting a low blood pressure is a far safer approach in the initial stages of resuscitation.

When I started at Noble's in 1990 there were three other consultants and four non-consultant anaesthetists, of which only two were experienced. Often, we had an anaesthetist or two who were either new to anaesthesia or had only one year's experience.

Today there are a total of sixteen anaesthetists and all are experienced – almost all are consultants. The workload now is therefore far less for each individual anaesthetist than it was thirty years ago. This means that the exposure of an individual anaesthetist to a particular situation is far less than it was years ago and it was something that often worried me. The result may be that the anaesthetist is less experienced at dealing with certain types of patients and therefore the care the patient receives may be of a lower standard than it might otherwise have been.

Today almost all general anaesthetics involve either the use of a tracheal tube, which is inserted with a laryngoscope, or a supraglottic airway device (SAD). Unlike the tube, this doesn't pass into the trachea, or windpipe. The anaesthetist's hands are freed up once a tube or SAD is in place.

The first time I used one of these was while working in Sunderland as a senior registrar in 1989. I remember working as a locum at Noble's for a couple of weeks during the TT festival that year and bringing some with me and demonstrating their use to Dougie Leece, the first time they had been used on the island.

When I started out the SAD hadn't been invented, so we would spend hours holding onto a face mask throughout the operation. After a few days my right hand would ache constantly, but within a few weeks this ceased as the muscles became stronger. The invention of the SAD, of which there are two main types, the Laryngeal Mask Airway (LMA) or the Igel, has had a serious downside in that the experience of managing the airway that we had when I started does not now exist. We would anaesthetise the patient then either intubate or hold onto a face mask. We'd learn little tricks for intubating or keeping even very difficult airways open during face mask anaesthetics.

Today, the facemask is only used for a very brief period, or even not at all, before the SAD is inserted. We would gain a lot of experience in intubating because far more patients were intubated than there are nowadays. Extensive use of the LMA or Igel means that many procedures which previously required a tube, are now done with these. The combined effect of this is that when a difficult airway is encountered the anaesthetist may be less equipped to deal with it, keep it open or intubate it.

Usually, when a tracheal tube was used, intubation was straightforward, but sometimes it could be difficult and on rare occasions impossible, due to variations in the anatomy of the airway in some patients. A bougie could often be passed into the trachea using the laryngoscope, then this could be used to guide the tube which was passed over it and railroaded into the trachea. Once the tube was felt to be correctly placed, the bougie would then be removed and the tube attached to the breathing system. A similar device, the intubating stylet, was used to stiffen the tube so it could be better directed during insertion. In the early days of my career this was all we had to help with difficult intubation. There are now many different types of laryngoscopes, videolaryngoscopes, fibreoptic flexible intubating scopes and a variety of other devices which may aid the anaesthetist. On occasion it still might prove impossible to pass the tube into the trachea.

Another factor which I feel has led to a deficit in modern training has come about due to the increasing use of regional anaesthesia – local anaesthetic techniques where the patient does not have a general anaesthetic.

Instead, local anaesthetic is injected around nerves supplying the area where the operation is to occur. For example, lower or upper limb surgery can be carried out under epidural or spinal anaesthesia, or by blocking nerves supplying the leg or arm. Patients who years ago would have needed a general anaesthetic for certain procedures can now have many operations without one. This has led to more lost opportunities for gaining experience with airway interventions. I'm not saying any of these developments are bad, I'm simply pointing out some consequences which have followed their introduction into anaesthesia.

I have actually heard very experienced ODPs voice similar concerns, worried about an anaesthetist. This, to me, is extremely worrying and raises serious questions about training in the specialty and the assessment of trainees' skills and the decision to sign them off as proficient and ready for the next stage of training, or their suitability for a consultant post where essentially they will be answerable to no one. If true, and there are deficits which have been overlooked during training, these inadequacies may only come to light in the event of a disaster in which a patient comes to some harm and they are revealed during the subsequent investigation or coroner's inquest into the incident. If the peers of an anaesthetist, anaesthetic colleagues and ODPs, have concerns, surely the best ones to be in a position to know, then some kind of action is needed. This could be a period of re-training, working under close supervision. There should also be feedback to those who signed the anaesthetist off in the first place as being proficient and an investigation into how this has come about.

In terms of actually administering a general anaesthetic, there have been too many changes during my career to mention here but one of the major ones involves the anaesthetic drugs themselves – the drugs keeping the patient unconscious during the operation. There are basically two types of general anaesthetic – inhalation or intravenous. With the former a short acting IV drug is usually given and once consciousness is lost, the rest of the anaesthetic continues with gas, usually air and oxygen with a volatile agent.

A volatile agent is an anaesthetic drug that is a liquid which evaporates quickly. The concentration is very carefully controlled by a vaporizer on the anaesthetic machine. The molecules in the vapour are the drugs which anaesthetise the patient and they are breathed in with air and added oxygen. This was always my preferred technique.

The other method of keeping a patient asleep is by Total Intravenous Anaesthesia (TIVA). The anaesthetic drugs are given intravenously during the anaesthetic by a continuous infusion through a syringe pump. This is a machine with a syringe containing the drug attached which delivers the drug at a carefully controlled rate into the IV line. It was in the early nineties when this started to gain popularity – when I started in 1983 it was rarely used by most anaesthetists. One surprising fact that as far as I'm aware hasn't changed, is that though there are several theories, we still don't know how anaesthetic drugs actually work in the brain.

There have been many developments in trying to make anaesthesia safer. Increased use of protocols for emergency treatment during an anaesthetic, various types of equipment for tracheal intubation in difficult cases and increased numbers of checklists prior to surgery are some examples. Some of the courses mentioned earlier would be thought to help reduce risk during surgery. For example, knowledge of the ALS (Advanced Life Support) should give an anaesthetist more confidence in dealing with a sudden arrhythmia during an operation. Improvements in monitoring equipment should help in earlier detection of problems arising in an anaesthetised patient.

If In Doubt

When I started pulse oximeters hadn't been invented. This device gives a continuous display of heart rate and the percentage of oxygen in the blood, the amount carried attached to haemoglobin in the red blood cells. I was having a chat in the office in the ICU at Arrowe Park Hospital in 1985 when I saw my first one. My young grandson goes to learn about first aid with St John's Ambulance and my daughter recently bought him a perfectly usable oximeter which clips onto a finger for ten pounds.

Before their use became the norm there were only two ways an anaesthetist really knew the patient was receiving an adequate amount of oxygen. By far the main one was simply by looking at their colour – if they were pink the patient would be thought to be adequately oxygenated. A slight bluish tinge was a very worrying sign. If there was any doubt the oxygen levels in the arterial blood had to be measured by taking an arterial sample and putting it through a blood gas analyser. It would take around ten to fifteen minutes to get the result.

Capnography is used for all patients who are being ventilated. This machine measures the amount of carbon dioxide the patient breathes out. If this level is high, ventilation is inadequate. In the Royal in Liverpool during my first year in 1983 there was one capnograph for the ten theatres and often there would be arguments over who got to use it.

Today few anaesthetists would give a general anaesthetic to a patient without attaching an oximeter and a capnograph. There would also be ECG monitoring and blood pressure measurement during the procedure. In spite of all of these measures – and this is my own view – I remain unconvinced that anaesthesia is any safer now than it was forty or fifty years ago. One of the reasons I say this is because general anaesthesia is very safe anyway. Years before I started there would be no ECG monitoring and blood pressure monitoring was often inaccurate. In spite of all of this, deaths due to anaesthesia even then were uncommon.

Many years ago, before I started my own career in anaesthesia, a common cause of a serious anaesthetic disaster which would cause death or hypoxic brain injury was a disconnection. Disconnection is defined as a break in continuity of the breathing circuit from an anaesthetic machine or ventilator to the patient's airway. There are several points where this can occur.

General anaesthesia as we know it today had its birth in the mid-19th century. For the first hundred years or so patients breathed spontaneously during the anaesthetic. In the 1940s, muscle relaxant drugs were introduced. These drugs allowed much lighter anaesthesia so patients woke up quicker. As they paralysed the abdominal muscles, they also made surgery easier. They also paralysed the breathing muscles, so patients had to be on a ventilator or manually ventilated by hand. The ventilator allowed the anaesthetist freedom of movement to perform his many other tasks, but in doing so, along with more and more elaborate surgical sterile draping of the patient, it had the effect of distancing the anaesthetist from the patient. If there had been a disconnection in a patient breathing spontaneously, the patient, instead of breathing anaesthetic gas and oxygen, would breathe air and start to wake up during surgery. If, however, this occurred in a ventilated patient, they would rapidly become hypoxic and suffer a cardiac arrest if the disconnection was not discovered.

Prior to ECG monitoring, blood pressure, pulse oximetry and capnography, the anaesthetist depended mainly on closely watching the breathing pattern, movement of the rubber bag, feeling a pulse and looking at the colour of the skin and at the pupils. With current monitoring, alarms sound when there is a disconnection. The sudden drop in pressure in the breathing system is detected by a ventilator alarm. The drop in oxygen levels

If In Doubt

detected by the oximeter and carbon dioxide by the capnograph both cause alarms to sound. The fall in heart rate due to low oxygen levels in the heart is detected by the ECG alarm.

I have always felt that no amount of expensive monitoring equipment is a substitute for constant vigilance by a well-trained anaesthetist when it comes to patient safety. 'The price of safety is eternal vigilance,' is a saying in anaesthesia. One of my consultant colleagues in the Isle of Man once told me a story I have never forgotten. Tony Rubin, one of his consultants at Charing Cross Hospital in London, told him during his training that the best monitor to ensure patient safety would be a three-foot-long chain. This would chain the anaesthetist to the operating table. If this actually existed it would prevent the anaesthetist from leaving the patient and potentially becoming distracted.

In an attempt to improve safety for patients by ensuring that all doctors working in the UK are up to scratch and make efforts to stay that way, there is now an established appraisal system in place. This is a major change not only for anaesthetists but for all doctors. It was a gradual process but is now a requirement for all. For the first fifteen years or so of my consultant post this didn't exist. An annual appraisal takes place for every doctor. Every five years the doctor will need to revalidate in order to continue to be able to practice.

He or she will need to demonstrate that they are reading journals and attending relevant courses and meetings to keep abreast of developments in their own specialty. Patient and colleague feedback needs to be collected so they can show that they are doing a reasonable job in the eyes of others. A surgeon must demonstrate they are doing a sufficient number of a particular type of operation to ensure they are maintaining their competency. The complaints officer for the hospital will give the doctor a letter saying how many, if any, complaints there have been in which the doctor has been named.

Reflection is an important part of the process. For example, if a mistake has been made this will be discussed during the appraisal meeting. The appraiser will want to see that lessons have been learnt and appropriate steps have been taken to reduce the risk in future and the doctor will hopefully have also informed colleagues so they can also learn from his mistake. Although, to me, it is far from a perfect process, the appraisal system can only be a good thing for patient care.

As I approached the thirtieth anniversary since starting in my consultant post I started to think about retirement. I'd often tell the ODPs I was worried I might make a serious mistake and I hoped I got out before anything like that happened. I still enjoyed the work and hadn't ever minded coming into the hospital in the middle of the night for emergency work. I'd been fortunate and never had a day's sick leave. I began to think about that anniversary and wondered whether that would be a good time to stop, after exactly thirty years in the post. My last day was to be June 30th 2020, a Tuesday.

I'd always wanted to tell the last patient I anaesthetised before stopping work that they would be the last. I have no idea why, but I'd often thought it would be a way to draw some imaginary line under what two thirds of my life had been. Including medical school, I'd been in medicine for almost forty-three years. I told a few colleagues this over the years and was talking to one a few days before I was due to retire.

'I hope you get a nice patient as your very last one,' she said.

It felt strange to think I'd not be giving any more anaesthetics ever again. The way I'd speak to patients on the wards before their operation and the things I'd say in the anaesthetic room over thirty-seven years had never really changed. I've never been sure why, but I never told any of them I was a doctor. I'd always introduce myself as Keith Wilkinson and tell them I was one of the anaesthetists and would be looking after them while they had their surgery. Sometimes, when they came into the anaesthetic room, they'd say, 'Hi Keith, how's it going?' or 'Alright Keith?' As soon as they lost consciousness the ODP, my assistant, would ask if they were a friend or did I know them. I'd say no; they'd assumed because they called me Keith I must have known them well. A lot of patients still don't know that anaesthetists are doctors.

As I'd be inserting the IV cannula, usually in the back of their hand, I'd always say,

'Just a little scratch coming up.' Now and then I'd add,

'I used to always say, "Just a little prick with a needle," until a few patients said, "Yeah, we all know you are, just get on with it will you?" I stopped saying it after that.'

That had never actually happened, but it usually got a laugh.

On Tuesday, my last day, I wasn't due to have an operating list. The day before that, my final day of clinical work, I was to cover theatre emergencies. There were no patients on my morning list. At lunchtime I was trying to find out about an incident involving a midwife and one of my colleagues and I wandered over to the obstetric ward. The midwife on the ward knew nothing about it and suggested I go into the labour ward as the two midwives there might be able to help me. As soon as I walked in two midwives took me by an arm each.

'Just the man!' one said, smiling. 'Come this way.'

They started to pull me towards a delivery room.

'Hang on, I'm only here to ask you something!'

'Never mind that, come in here.'

If In Doubt

In the room a patient was in labour, using gas and air as a contraction started. One of the midwives explained that one of my colleagues had inserted an epidural but it wasn't working. They'd asked him about it but he'd said he was sure it was in the right place and he couldn't do any more. He was also then about to start a caesarean section. I spoke to her and it was clear that there was no effect at all from the epidural. She needed another one. As I was doing the epidural I said to her this would be my last epidural ever after several thousand over a thirty-five-year period. A midwife asked what I meant by that. I told her that the following day would be my last. She looked shocked.

'You can't leave!' she said.

'We're going to start a petition to stop you leaving!'

The epidural was working well and I left to see the only patient on my afternoon list. When I heard what he was having I was a bit disappointed. My colleague had said she hoped I got a nice final patient. It appeared this wasn't going to be the case. He had a fractured mandible (a fractured jaw). Invariably these patients have been in a drunken fight. I went to the ward to see him. He was sitting on the edge of the bed, muscular and covered in tattoos. I asked him what had happened.

'I was fighting a lad I used to train with when we were boxers.'

'Are the police involved?' I enquired. He said no, they weren't. The other man had rang him and apologised and there were no hard feelings.

An hour or so later we were in the anaesthetic room. As I was putting the cannula I said it.

'I think you are going to be the last patient I ever anaesthetise.'

It took about an hour to insert metal plates to fix the fractured bone. I saw him as he was coming round in the recovery ward and he fist bumped me and insisted we had

If In Doubt

our photo taken together. A colleague took it. I had been lucky after all; he was a nice guy.

Although I'd insisted I wanted nothing on my last day, at five o'clock many of my colleagues from around the hospital were in the lecture theatre of the Education Centre to say their goodbyes. I said a few words about my career and was presented with a laminated photo showing me with my last patient, who had written a few words wishing me well. For me it was the perfect ending. Earlier that afternoon I'd arranged to have an email sent to everyone in the hospital as a way of saying goodbye:

Hi all,

I started officially as a consultant anaesthetist at Noble's exactly 30 years ago tomorrow, 1st July 1990. I also started my career as a doctor on the island in July 1982 after training in Liverpool, working as a house officer for a year here and deciding then I was going to be an anaesthetist. Three months after I started, in October 1982 I met Kerry at a doctors' party in the old hospital and we were married at the end of Race Week in June 1983.

During my training back in Liverpool and then Newcastle I did locums in anaesthetics on the island during TT fortnight, so I think I've actually done some work every year here for 38 years.

During my whole career I've been very lucky – I've never been off sick and never once woke up and thought I didn't want to go to work. I've enjoyed every minute although there have been some stressful and upsetting times along the way too. I feel very privileged to have been able to do the job I've done. I'd like to thank everyone I've worked with, especially the nurses and midwives who I've always felt do a fantastic job but don't always get the credit they deserve for an often difficult and stressful job. Thanks to the ODPs for always 'having my back!' We are very lucky to have our lovely three daughters and six – soon to be seven – beautiful grandchildren all here and settled on the island; the oldest is nine.

I'd like to wish everyone who knows me all the best for the future and thank you all for making my time working here so enjoyable. I know I'm going to miss the social side of work and especially the clinical work. It seems to me that it has almost become a 'Manx tradition' that when people leave the hospital, maybe have a 'leaving do'– or even three – and say goodbye it is almost guaranteed they will be back again very soon. I'd be a hypocrite if I also did this as I've never understood it so if anyone does see me wandering around the hospital, probably carrying my guitar, would they please tell me off!

Best wishes to everyone,
Keith

As I'd anxiously awaited the arrival of the consultant surgeon on the day I'd started work on the Isle of Man as a house officer on July 26th 1982, I'd thought, 'I hope I'll be good enough.' Now, as I walked out of the hospital as an anaesthetist for the last time that evening, almost thirty-eight years later, I had another thought - 'I hope I was.'

ACKNOWLEDGEMENTS

Many people have helped me write this book. I'd like to thank them all - my daughters, friends and ex-colleagues at the hospital who have happily read occasional chapters and given me their honest opinion. I'd also like to thank numerous others who have given valuable feedback on my efforts to explain medical procedures in a way that will hopefully be easily understood by a lay person.

I want to express particular gratitude to Diane Butler, who used to be the anaesthetic secretary at Noble's Hospital. I want her to know how much I value her honesty. As well as Diane, I owe a lot to copywriter Jacqueline Morrey-Grace, who also lives on the Isle of Man, for all her help and advice, and my middle daughter Katie, an English teacher. I have told Katie and Jackie that they are 'proper writers' and I'm just an amateur in comparison. There is no doubt that the quality of the book has been enhanced by the support I have had from all three.

The clinical scenarios I describe throughout the book are all true and are based on real patients and real events. I have, however, anonymised them to maintain patient confidentiality. Although they will never know that they feature in my book I want to thank them all anyway.

Finally, I want to say a big thank you to Jennie Hunter for her kind foreword, and the team at New Generation Publishing for their patience, courtesy and professionalism in helping me to publish this book, in particular, David Walshaw, Saskia Osterloff and Nick Roberts for the cover design.

Printed in Great Britain
by Amazon